manalivinghealing.com

Copyright © 2021 Vera Powles

All rights reserved. No part of this book may be reproduced or used in any manner without the prior written permission of the copyright owner, except for the use of brief quotations in a book review.

Although the author and publisher have made every effort to ensure that the information in this book was correct at press time, the author and publisher do not assume and hereby disclaim any liability to any party for any loss, damage, or disruption caused by errors or omissions, whether such errors or omissions result from negligence, accident, or any other cause.

This book is not intended to be a substitute for the medical advice of a licensed physician. The reader should consult with their doctor in any matters relating to their health.

Paperback: 9798756650501

Hardcover: 9798756694048

First edition: November 2021.

Edited by Stephanie Clements

Layout by Alfiyan (LaunchBetterCo)

Acknowledgements

A huge thank you to Stephanie Clements who reviewed and edited this book. I'm so grateful for your patience, kindness, impeccable sense of humour and for all the time we got to spend together recently.

I grew up watching my, very talented, mum Cila catering for parties whilst, with all the patience in the world, she instilled a love for cooking in me. Despite all the hardship she's been through, she always made me believe I could do anything I set my mind to and has supported me unconditionally throughout my life.

I would not have been able to write this book without my husband's support and encouragement. Thank you for growing with me and making me feel loved, every single day.

Thank you to all my friends and clients for your enthusiasm and courageously testing some of the recipes in this book.

Hi there,

I'm Vera - an Integrative Nutrition Health Coach and Women's Circles Leader. Using my background in Molecular Medicine allied to my holistic nutrition certification and experience coaching clients on their health transformations, I have developed a framework called Six Pillars of Wellness.

A healthy state goes beyond the absence of illness. It is a combination of physical, mental, spiritual and emotional wellbeing so I truly believe in a holistic approach to wellness which integrates the whole being.

Research in the area of genetics (1,2) strongly suggests that positive lifestyle changes can impact our predisposition to certain diseases. So my aim with this programme is to give your body the best opportunity possible to heal whilst easily sustaining your new habits.

Thank you for trusting me on this journey and taking the first step towards making yourself a priority.

In love and gratitude, always

Vera x

manalivinghealing.com

vera.powles

facebook.com/
manalivinghealing

manalivinghealing
@gmail.com

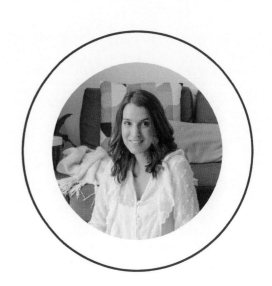

Contents

The Mana Living Mindset

Set Yourself Up for Success

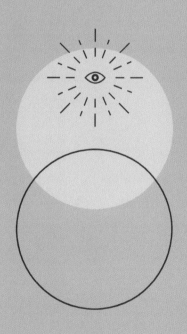

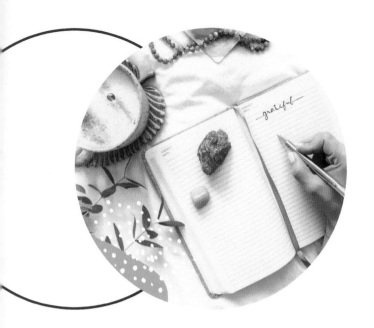

The Mana Living Mindset

We all know we should be eating lots of greens, exercising regularly and sleeping well, so why do we struggle so much in doing it consistently? There are many different layers to this question but, for me, it all comes down to the systems you have in place.

What I see time and time again with my clients is that, we tend to focus on the goal itself, on what we want to achieve, without carefully planning how we will get there. Willpower will help you take the first step, but it's your strategy that will help you became who you want to be (3).

This is the essence of this book; I will give you the tools you need to build a strategy that works for you and is sustainable. I'll present different habit building tips throughout the book which you can experiment with, to find what best suits you as an individual.

I'll invite you to read through the book first and get familiar with the importance of these 3 pillars of wellbeing: diet, exercise and sleep. The last chapter will help you put together all you have learned and design new, structured habits that serve your lifestyle. By being specific and planning ahead, you can take the fatigue out of the decision making process and eliminate barriers to the creation of new habits.

Although this is a programme, the aim here is not to lose a certain amount of weight or look a certain way. Once the 30 days are over, I want you to feel inspired, stronger and happier about yourself, as well as feeling confident that you can carry on your newfound lifestyle forever.

Instead of seeing this as a health-kick, I want you to think of this programme as the first step to a new way of living. A lifestyle in which you will be free from diet culture, have a renewed vitality, a fresh mindset and improved mental health.

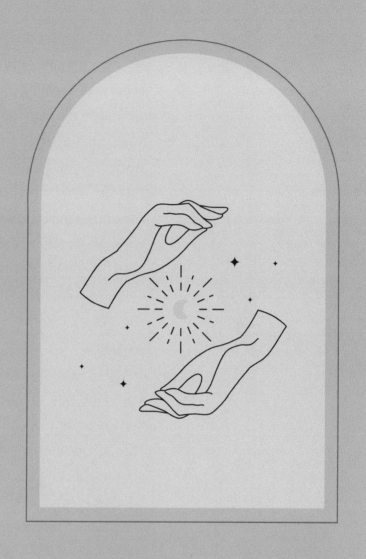

Building Awareness

We Can Only Change What We Know

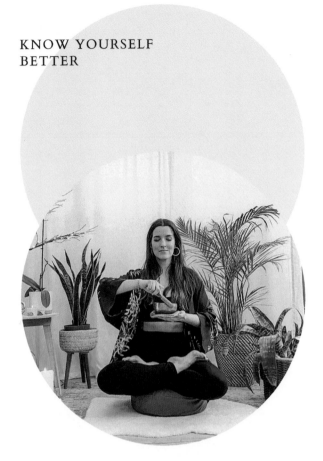

Building Awareness

*We can only manage
what we monitor*

Before we move onto the fun part, let us begin with knowing yourself better.

We move through life a million miles an hour, but how often do we sit down to take stock of our life, habits and happiness?

This is what this chapter is about - knowing where you are right now, so you know where to focus your attention for the next 30 days. I'm a firm believer in bioindividuality meaning there is no one-size fits all approach when it comes to wellness.

So while the programme might be the same, the way we approach it will largely depend on your routine and lifestyle.

Throughout these next pages you'll assess your levels of happiness across each of my 6 Pillars of Wellness. This will allow you to know which areas of your life might be interfering with your ability to form healthy habits and explore the root cause of this.

Since habit change is such an important part of this book, you'll also complete an introspection exercise to gauge how your priorities align with your current actions.

Circle of Life

Place a dot within each segment to indicate your level of satisfaction in each pillar of your life.

A dot towards the centre indicates dissatisfaction, and a dot towards the periphery indicates satisfaction. So the closer your dot is to the periphery, the happier you are with that area of your life. Then, connect the dots to see your Circle of Life (adapted from the Institute for Integrative Nutrition).

Now that we have identified imbalances, we can determine where to spend more time and energy to improve it.

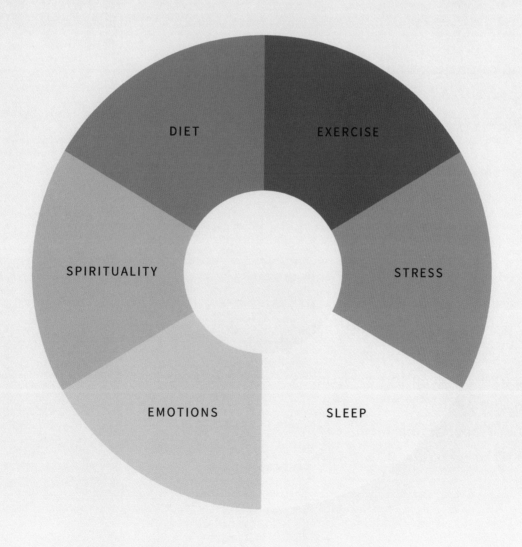

Are You Living In Alignment?

Write down up to five priorities regarding your wellbeing (you can add less if you want).
e.g. having a mindful morning routine

See if you can match a current habit to each priority. Ask yourself: "what behaviours, if any, align with my goals?"
e.g. I wake up at 06:30 every morning which gives me 1h before work

Then assess if you have a current habit which is working against that priority. Ask yourself: "what behaviours are preventing me from reaching my goals?"
e.g. I spend too much time mindlessly scrolling on social media as soon as I wake up

Now that we have identified the imbalances in your life and the barriers to your healthy habits, it's time to let go of what is not serving you. If you want lasting results you need to reset the habits that no longer align with the person you want to become.

If we were to discuss our habits, they would likely look different from person to person. However, one thing they would all have in common is that we can break them down into steps as follows (3):

- It all starts with a <u>Reminder</u> (e.g. you wake up and walk to the bathroom)
- Then comes the <u>Response</u> to (e.g. you brush your teeth)
- And finally, the <u>Reward</u> (e.g. a clean mouth)

Research shows that, if one of these steps fail, you cannot build a habit. Similarly, if you want to change an existing habit you need to be aware of the Response but also the Reminder (4). Unless we develop full consciousness and awareness of our habits, we won't succeed at changing them (4).

Throughout this book, I'll provide suggestions for successful habit change. As a start, reflect on whether any of these strategies would work for you and how you can implement them, even before you start the programme:

1. **Monitoring** (5): we tend to overestimate our positive habits and underestimate our less helpful ones. In chapter six, "The Programme", you'll find a variety of trackers which you can use to monitor your progress and happiness.
2. **Scheduling** (4, 6): eliminating the decision making process in everyday choices can improve the chances of sticking to healthy habits. At the start of each week, if you schedule all your workouts, plan your meals and set up reminders to go to bed you'll find it easier to start a routine that favours habit formation. Chapter six includes planners and action plans that will make scheduling easier. You might also find some <u>helpful videos</u> on my Instagram account.
3. **Accountability** (4, 6): for some people, monitoring and scheduling will act like accountability in itself. For others, further external accountability might be needed, so let someone else know you're doing this programme, or even better, find a programme partner to help keep you on track. Join the <u>Facebook Group</u> (see page 89) to find an accountability partner and be inspired by others' progress.

Your lifestyle should be more than what you do. It should be who you are!

#manalivinghealing

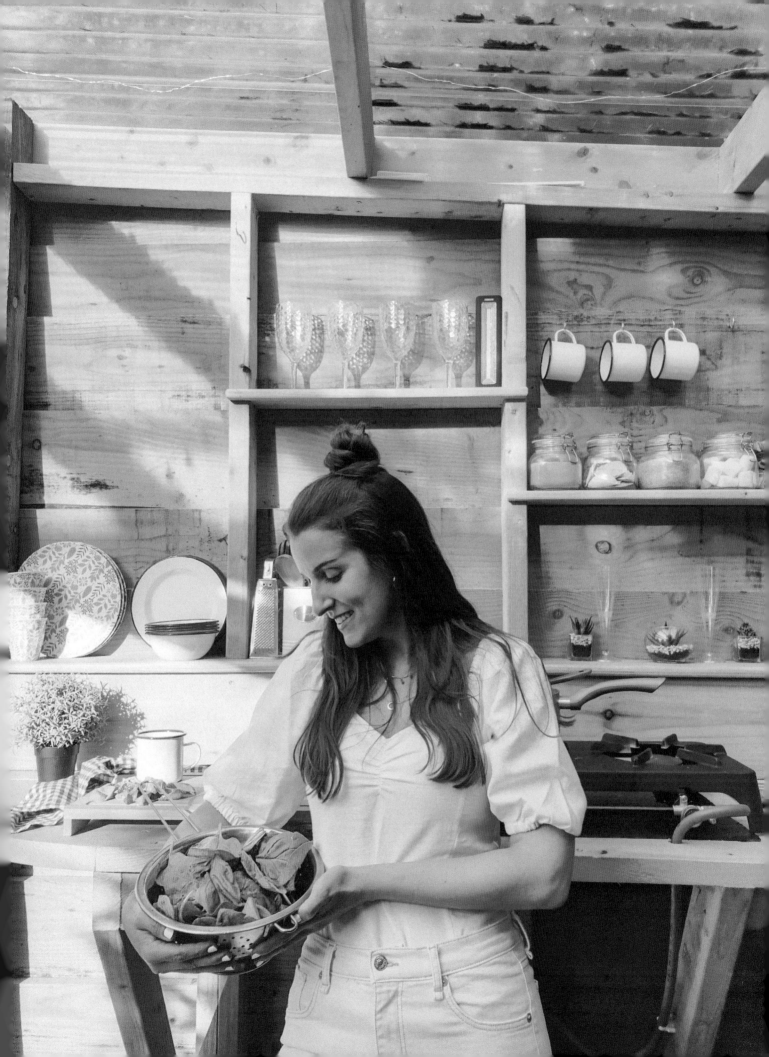

Eat Well

Find Nourishment and Enjoyment In Food

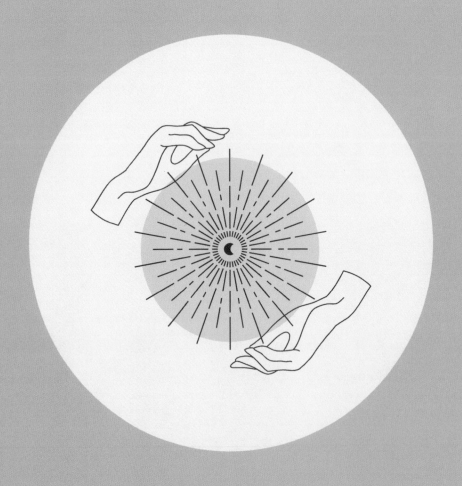

Eat Well

I believe that diet is one of the foundations of wellbeing so, unsurprisingly, it's an important part of this programme.

Eating well doesn't have to be complicated! In essence, it means returning to a whole, unrefined diet filled with fresh fruit, vegetables and whole, unprocessed grains. I don't believe in highly restrictive diets or calorie counting. So in this programme, there's no focus on the amount of food you eat but rather the quality of it.

I put an emphasis on natural, whole, plant based foods due to mounting evidence of how they act to prevent chronic disease, cancer and inflammation in the body (7).

The plate on the right is how I strive to eat everyday to feel satiated and full of vitality. Nutrition is highly individual so feel free to use the plate as a guide and adapt it to what feels best for your body. Around the plate there is a larger circle demonstrating the importance of proper hydration throughout the day, as well as non-dietary aspects of our lives.

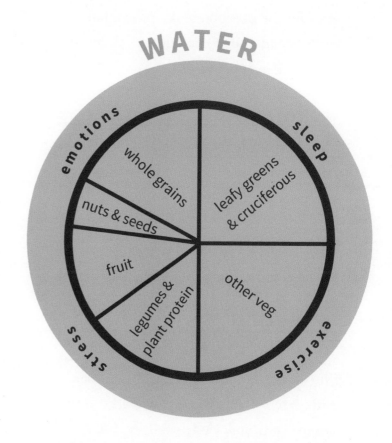

This is because the lack of coping mechanisms for daily stressors (8), inconsistent exercise habits, poor sleep and emotional regulation can impact our diet. These non-dietary aspects can be complex triggers behind poor dietary habits (9).

For example, if the diet habits that are not serving you are rooted in emotional eating, you need to address this holistically. Until you have worked on your emotions, it's unlikely you will be able to sustain your diet changes.

Of course, in life there should always be space for the occasional indulgence but, at least for the duration of the programme, I recommend you try to cut out as much processed food as you can.

These are usually highly addictive foods so it's important to loosen the grip they have on you if you want to use this programme to change your habits.

If you follow the layout of the plate on the previous page, there isn't much space for processed food and you'll naturally crowd these out from your diet.

The recipes on the next pages are packed with the vitamins, minerals and antioxidants your body needs to feel and function at its best.

They have also been designed to allow for preparation of larger quantities which can be eaten throughout the week, very much like my usual meal prep.

Before the start of each week write down which meals you'll have each day for breakfast, lunch and dinner. Prepare or cook these on a Sunday so you have a fridge full of ready-to-eat food, allowing you more time to spend on yourself without feeling overwhelmed. Although it might sound challenging, please give it a try. I see much better success rates in clients who can incorporate meal prep in their weekly routine.

Throughout the programme try and drink two litres of water everyday. We wake up dehydrated so have a large glass (500ml) of warm water with a slice of lemon first thing in the morning.

Eating well changes your consciousness. If you meditate every day but then eat a family-sized bucket of KFC that'll only take you so far.

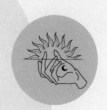

Breakfast

My Favourite Smoothies

Ingredients

Espresso & PB

- 200ml plant based milk
- 1 frozen banana
- 1 shot of espresso or decaf
- 1tbsp peanut butter
- 1tbsp oats
- 1tbsp milled flaxseed
- 1tsp maca (optional)

Greens & Mango

- 200ml plant based milk
- a handful of baby spinach
- a handful of chopped kale
- 1 cup frozen mango
- 1tbsp milled flaxseed
- 1tbsp hemp seeds
- 1tsp spirulina

Berry & Orange

- 150ml plant based milk
- juice of 1 orange
- 1 cup frozen mixed berries
- 1tbsp milled flaxseed
- 1tbsp hemp seeds
- 2 tbsp of your favourite plant based yoghurt

Prep: **10** m   Servings: **1**

Directions

01   Place all ingredients in a blender and blend until smooth.

02   Adjust the consistency by adding more plant based milk if needed.

Note: If you want to make a more substantial smoothie just add 2tbsp oats or 1tbsp of nut butter before blending. If you need a little sweetness add 1tsp of maple syrup.

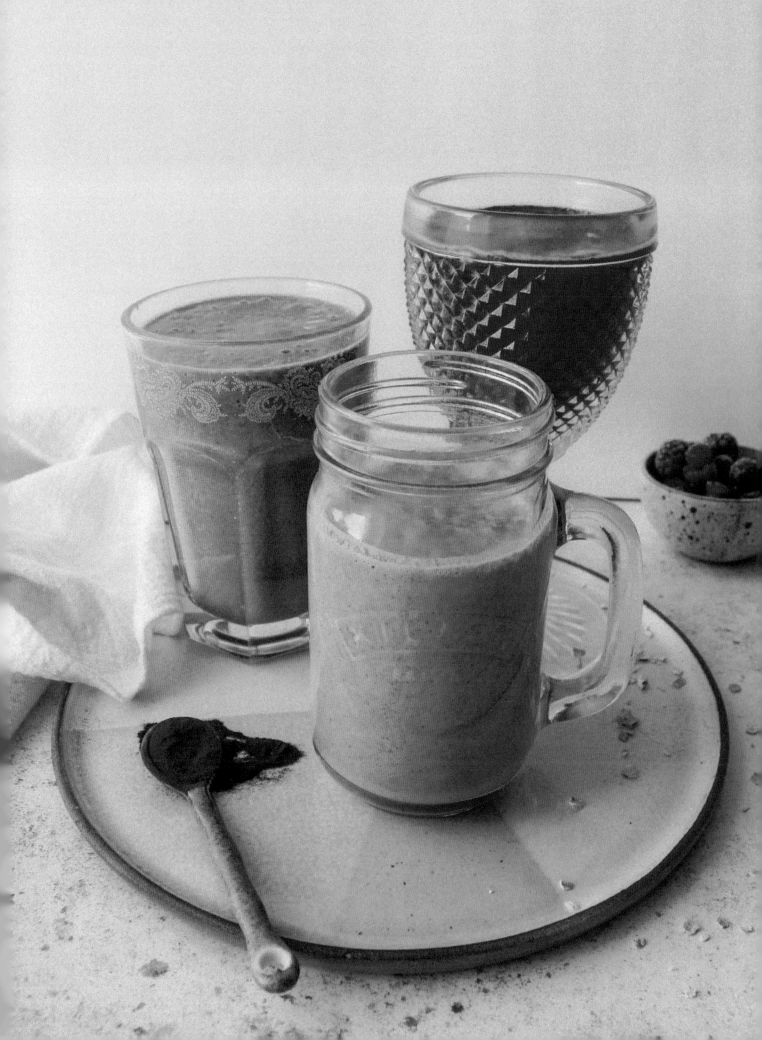

Sriracha Butter

Ingredients

- 200g cashew nuts
- 4tsp Sriracha
- 1tbsp coconut oil, melted
- 1tbsp nutritional yeast
- 1tsp garlic powder
- 1tsp salt
- 1tsp freshly ground pepper

Prep: **10** m (+ soaking)   Servings: **makes 250ml**

Directions

01   Soak the cashew nuts for 6 hours or overnight. If you have a really powerful blender (I use a NutriBullet) a couple of hours in hot water might suffice.

02   Drain the cashew nuts. Add all ingredients to a food processor and blend until you have a super smooth cream. If needed, add a splash of water.

03   Store in an airtight jar in the fridge.

Note: This "butter" elevates even the simplest dish. I love it over the Spicy Sweet Potatoes on page 52. Cashew nuts are high in protein, a good source of magnesium and are suggested to reduce the risk of heart disease.

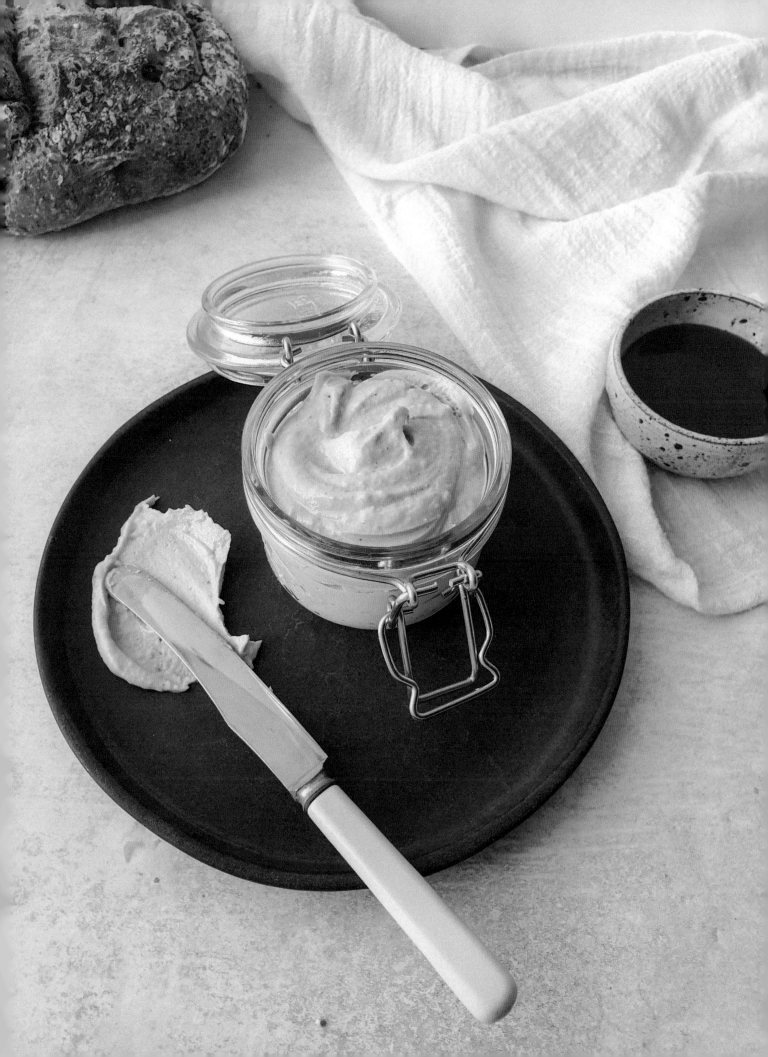

The Best Avocado Toast

Ingredients

- 1 slice of your favourite bread (I love rye sourdough)
- 1tsp mixed herbs (I think coriander and chives work particularly well here)
- 1/2 avocado
- 2tsp of Sriracha butter (page 20)
- a pinch of salt
- freshly ground black pepper
- 1tbsp seed mix (sesame, sunflower, linseed, etc.)
- a handful of rocket

Prep: **5** m Servings: **1**

Directions

01 Put the bread to toast. Chop the herbs. Remove the pit and scoop the flesh out of the avocado. Thinly slice.

02 Spread the sriracha butter on the toasted bread. Add the avocado slices and season with salt and pepper.

03 Top with the herbs, seeds and rocket.

Note: Avocado toast is my favourite breakfast ever! I've spent years perfecting it and this is my favourite combination. It's also full of healthy fats, which will keep you satiated until lunch and ensure proper brain function.

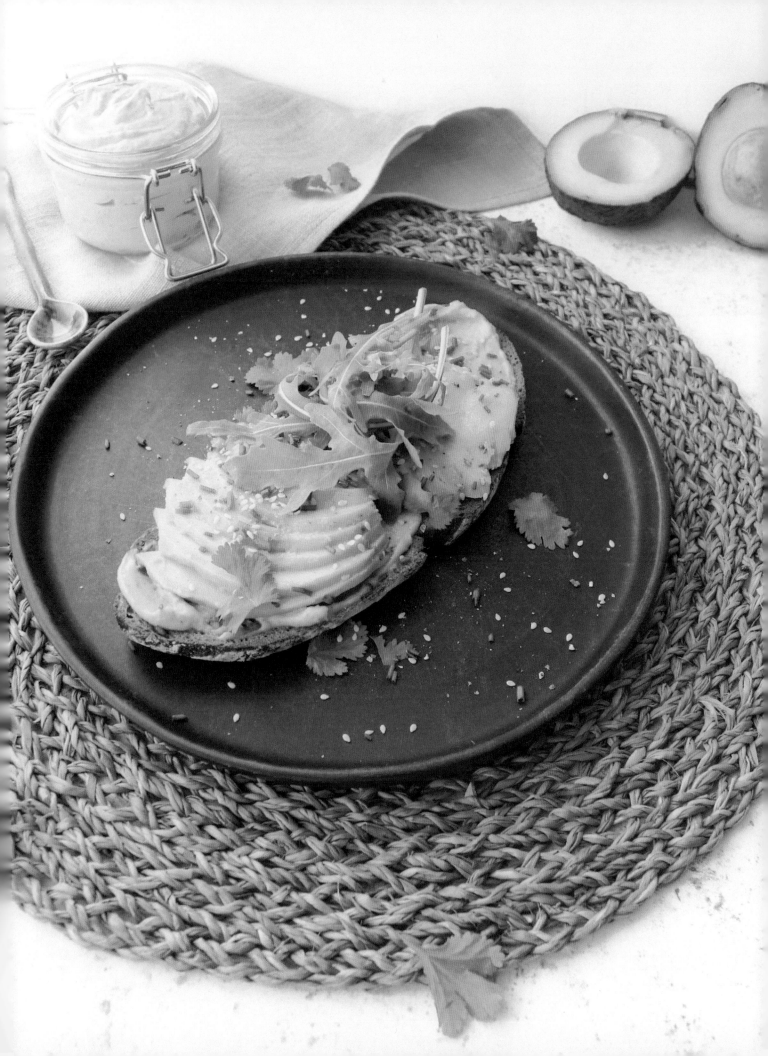

Mana Living Granola

Ingredients

Prep: **10** m Cook: **35** m Servings: **14**

- 350g oats
- 1 cup coconut oil
- 100g macadamia nuts
- 80g dried mango
- 40g sunflower seeds
- 50g pumpkin seeds
- 1/2 cup maple syrup
- 100g coconut chips

Directions

01 Preheat your oven to 160°C. Melt the coconut oil. Roughly chop the macadamia nuts and mango pieces if they are too big.

02 In a large bowl, mix in the oats, seeds, chopped nuts, melted coconut oil and maple syrup. Mix well.

03 Line a large baking sheet with greaseproof paper and distribute the granola evenly (you might need to spread it across 2 different baking sheets). Bake for 30 minutes, stirring every 10 minutes to ensure it cooks evenly.

04 Remove from the oven, stir in the coconut chips and chopped mango and return to the oven for another 5 minutes.

05 Remove from the oven and let it cool at room temperature before storing in an airtight container. Keeps for several weeks.

Note: the time I spent in Hawai'i had such a life-changing impact on me, it was only fair to name this exotic granola after my favourite Hawaiian word (which also just happens to be the name of my brand).

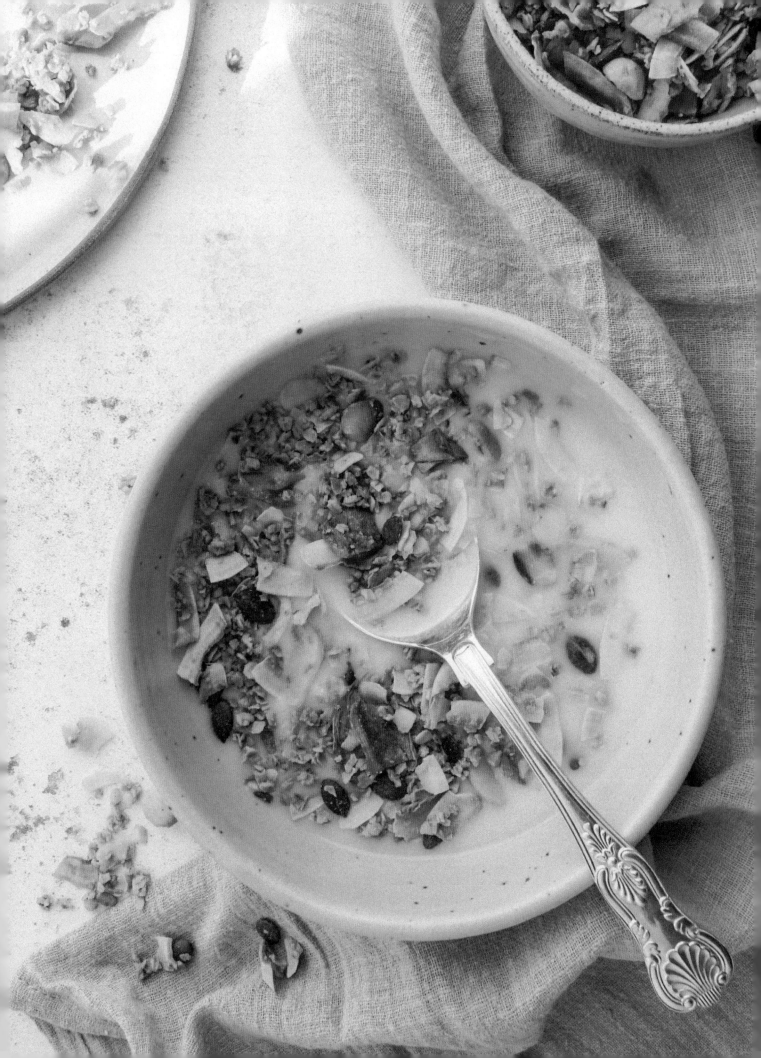

Yoghurt Bowl

Ingredients

- 1 banana
- 1/2tsp coconut oil
- 1tsp maple syrup
- 175g coconut yoghurt (or other plant-based yoghurt, preferably with live cultures)
- a handful of blueberries
- a handful of strawberries
- 1tbsp milled flaxseed
- 1tbsp of your favourite seed mix (I love a mix of hemp seeds, goldenberries, mulberries, cacao nibs and goji berries)
- 1/2tsp ground cinnamon

Directions

01   Slice the banana. In a small frying pan, on medium heat, add the coconut oil until it's melted followed by the maple syrup. Fry the bananas a couple of minutes each side until they are golden and caramelised.

02   Halve or quarter the strawberries.

02   To a small bowl add the plant-based yoghurt and top it with the caramelised banana, berries, flaxseed, seed mix and cinnamon.

Note: You can vary the fruits according to what's in season; figs, caramelised apples and berry compote or papaya, mango and passion fruit are some of my favourites.

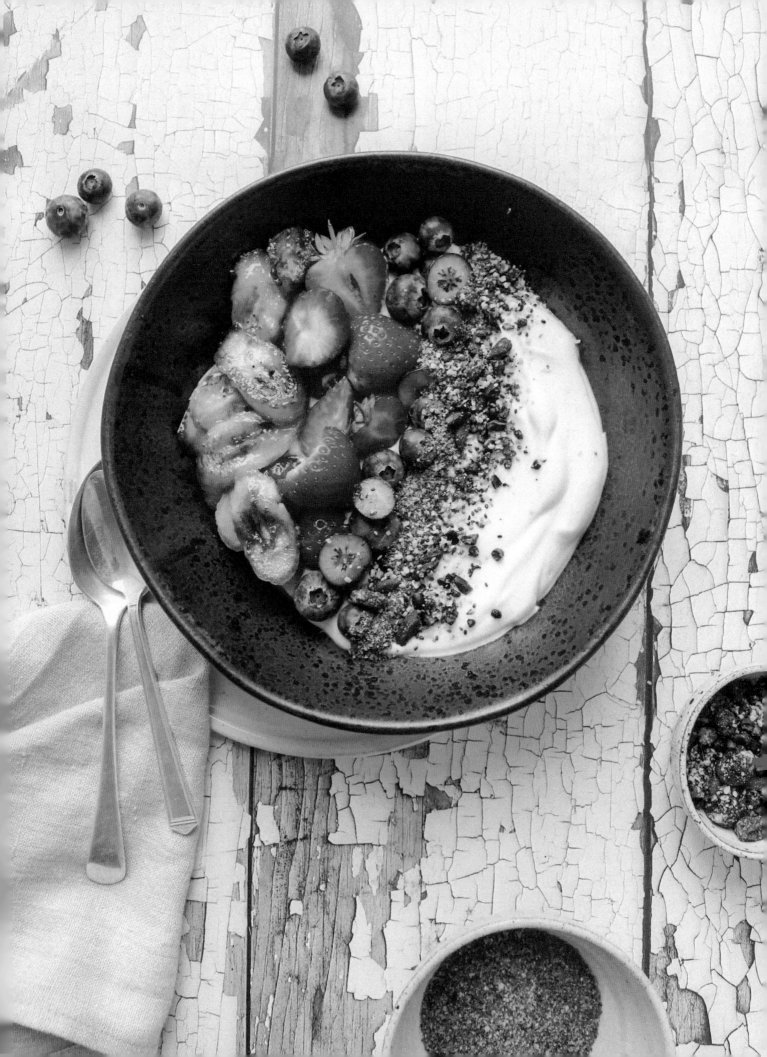

Mini Tofu Frittatas

Ingredients

- 1 small onion
- 9 sundried tomatoes
- 2 to 3tbsp black olives, pitted
- 1tbsp chives
- 1tbsp flat leaf parsley
- 1tbsp olive oil
- 120g spinach
- 280g firm tofu
- 1/2 cup almond milk
- 1tbsp nutritional yeast
- 1/4tsp turmeric
- 1/2tsp garlic powder
- 1/2tbsp cornstarch
- salt & freshly ground pepper

Note: These mini frittatas are so versatile - they make a brilliant breakfast or brunch, go really well in a lunch box or as part of a picnic spread.

Prep: **15** m   Cook: **30** m   Servings: **9**

Directions

01 Pre-heat the oven to 180°C. Chop the onion finely, dice the sundried tomatoes and slice the olives. Finely chop the chives and parsley.

02 Heat the olive oil in a non-stick frying pan. Add the chopped onion and cook on a medium heat until translucent without allowing to brown. Then add the sundried tomatoes and olives. Cook for a minute before adding the spinach. Cook until wilted. Season well with salt and pepper.

03 To a food processor, add the tofu (roughly broken into pieces), almond milk, nutritional yeast, turmeric, garlic powder, cornstarch, salt and pepper. Blend until you get a smooth, uniform mixture.

04 Stir the cooked veg into the tofu mixture and add in the parsley and chives.

05 Lightly grease a muffin tray and scoop the mixture into each cup - you should have enough for 9. Bake for 30 minutes.

06 Once baked, leave to cool for 15 minutes. To remove from the muffin tray, run a knife around the edges of each muffin cup and carefully lift each mini frittata.

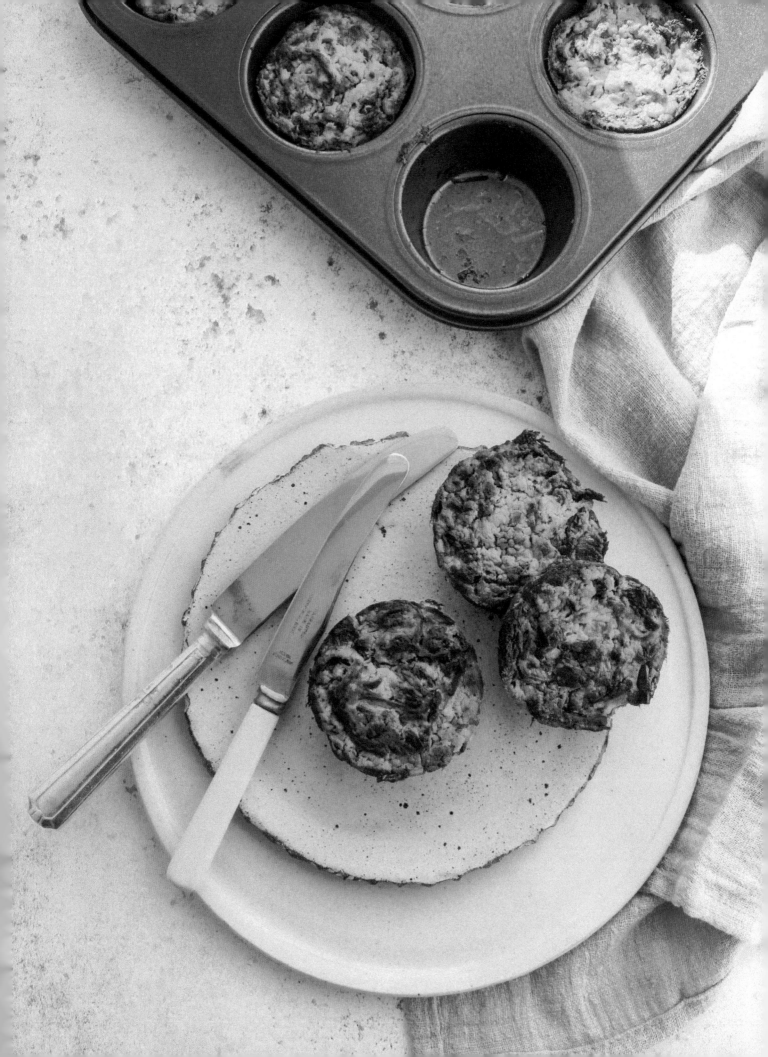

Mana refers to the life force we cannot see but is present in all things. It is spiritual energy as well as healing power. It comes from knowing who you are, where you come from and what your life purpose is.

#manalivinghealing

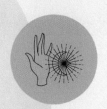

Meal Prep

A Note
On Meal Prep

You will have seen photos of meal preps on social media which consist of multiple food storage containers with identical contents. That's not what I mean by Meal Prep here.

The way we'll do meal prep is by preparing different components (from our Plate on page 16) which you can mix and match each day, as if you had a deli in your fridge. There are two main reasons I do it this way; variety and fatigue.

When you prepare 10 containers of tofu, broccoli and rice, you'll receive the nutrients of these ingredients only for the entire week. It's still healthy but it's not very balanced because you're lacking diversity. You're also more likely to suffer from food fatigue.

If, by Thursday evening, you have already had 6 portions of the same food, you are more likely to order a take away or run to the supermarket for convenience food to add some diversity. Not only will it not be as healthy, but you'll be wasting food, your time and money.

The idea is not to prepare huge, time consuming recipes but instead, several quick and simple side dishes you can combine for different meals throughout the week.

Meal prepping can seem like an intimidating and lengthy process, but I promise it will save you time and bring flexibility to your week. Be clever with the timings - I prepare everything for the oven first, in the meantime I cook things on the hob and whilst that happens, I make any salads and dressings. As you meal prep week after week, you'll find your flow and it'll become easier and quicker.

On the next page, you'll find a cheatsheet guide on what to prepare ahead of each week. This guide covers lunch and dinner for two people over five days, so adjust it according to your lifestyle and needs.

Prep For Success Cheatsheet
My typical meal prep for a week's worth of meals for two people

1 batch (around 500g) of wholegrains
brown rice, wholemeal pasta, quinoa, barley, etc.
simply cooked or as a salad mixed with beans, veggies and/or herbs

3x plant-based protein / beans
tofu, tempeh, chickpeas, lentils, beans, etc.
as bean salads, stews, falafel or bean patties

1x cruciferous
broccoli, cauliflower, Brussels sprouts, cabbage, etc.
simply steamed, roasted with spices, finely chopped in a slaw

2x leafy greens
kale, rocket, spinach, chard, watercress, etc.
as a salad, tossed in pasta or mixed with beans and/or other veggies

2x (or more) other veggies
squash, mushrooms, beetroot, peppers, sweet potatoes, etc.
roasted, raw, in a marinade, sautéed or as a salsa

2x dip or sauce
using nuts, beans, veggies or spices (e.g. harissa), dips or a simple
vinaigrette are a great way of adding more nutrients and changing the
flavour of your meals throughout the week

MEAL

PREP

Super Rice

Ingredients

Prep: **10** m   Cook: **40** m   Servings: **4** m

- 70g brown basmati rice
- 20g quinoa
- 2tbsp extra virgin olive oil
- 200g shiitake mushrooms
- 300g cauliflower, made into rice in a food processor
- 1tsp miso paste
- 2 garlic cloves, minced
- freshly ground black pepper

Directions

01   Cook the brown rice and quinoa according to the package instructions.

02   Dice the mushrooms. Cut the cauliflower into florets and add to a food processor. Pulse until it turns into cauliflower rice.

03   Heat the olive oil in a large frying pan or wok on medium heat (don't let it smoke!). Add the shiitake mushrooms and cook, undisturbed for 3 minutes or until golden. Give them a stir and cook for another 3 minutes.

04   Add the miso paste and garlic and cook for a minute (add a little water if needed). Add the cauliflower rice and sauté for 5 to 8 minutes and season well with the pepper.

05   Once the brown rice and quinoa are cooked, drain well and add to the frying pan. Stir until everything is well combined.

Note: A nutrition bomb - rich in protein, fibre and B vitamins, these ingredients support your cardiovascular health, immune system and are full of phytonutrients that can protect against cancer.

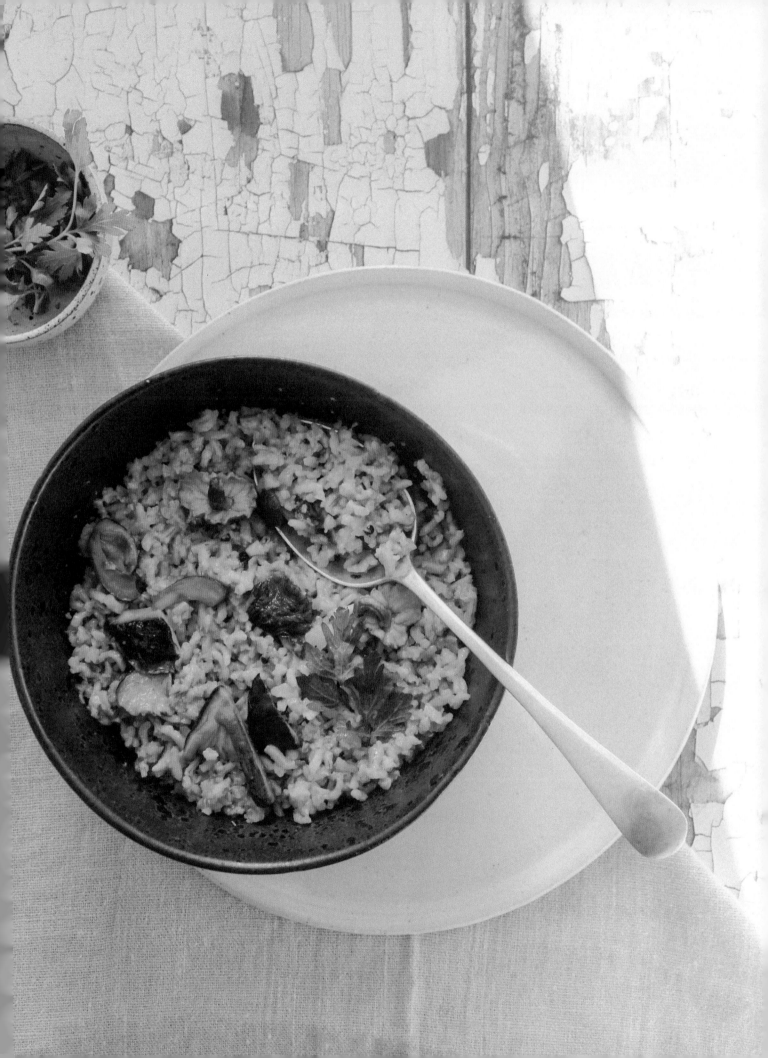

Tomato & "Mascarnone" Pasta

Ingredients

- 80g cashew nuts
- 250g cherry tomatoes
- 3 cloves of garlic
- 3tbsp olive oil
- 300g red lentil penne (or your favourite pasta)
- 3tbsp tomato paste
- 1/2tsp smoked paprika
- a squeeze of lemon juice
- 1tbsp nutritional yeast
- salt & freshly ground pepper
- a handful of basil leaves (optional)

Note: This pasta works really well on its own with sautéed mushrooms and spinach or as a side with the Simple Garlic & Chilli Greens on page 50 and the Herby Tofu on page 38.

Directions

01 Soak the cashew nuts for 6 hours or overnight. If you have a really powerful blender (I use a NutriBullet) a couple of hours in hot water might suffice.

02 Pre-heat your oven to 200ºC. Boil a kettle. Halve the cherry tomatoes. Place the halved tomatoes, cut-side up, and the garlic cloves (skin on) in a roasting tray. Drizzle with 2tbsp of olive oil and season with salt and pepper. Pop in the oven for 20 minutes or until the skin is blistered and slightly charred. Once roasted, remove from the oven and set aside.

03 Cook the pasta according to the packaging instructions. Drain once cooked and reserve the cooking water.

04 Drain the cashew nuts and add to a food processor together with the roasted tomatoes, peeled roasted garlic, tomato paste, smoked paprika, lemon juice, nutritional yeast, 60ml water, 1tbsp olive oil, salt and pepper. Blend until creamy, adding more water if needed. Toss into the pasta adding some of the cooking water to loosen it up. Serve with torn basil leaves and freshly ground pepper.

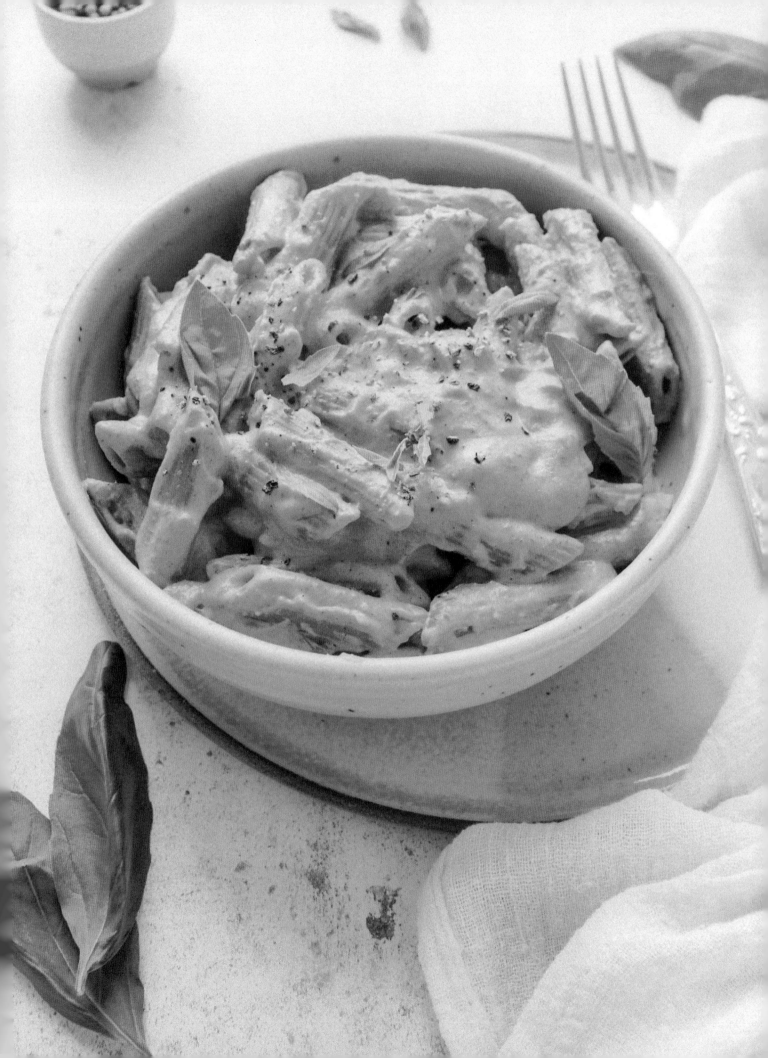

Tofu, 3 Ways

These are my favourite ways of eating tofu. The Herby Tofu is great eaten cold, and both the Harissa and Scrambled Tofu taste better heated up.

Herby Tofu

Ingredients

- 300g super firm tofu (preferably organic)
- 60ml extra-virgin olive oil
- juice of 1 lemon
- 1tsp Dijon mustard
- 10g parsley, finely chopped
- 10g chives, finely chopped
- 5g dill, finely chopped
- 2 garlic cloves, bashed
- salt and pepper, to taste

Prep: **10** min (+ marinating)   Cook: **10** min   Servings: 4

Directions

01 Drain the tofu block and press it using a clean tea towel or kitchen paper to remove as much moisture as you can. Cut the tofu into 8 equal slices.

02 Heat a griddle pan over medium heat and, once hot, add the tofu. You might need to cook in batches so the tofu slices don't touch each other. Cook each side for 5 minutes undisturbed or until the tofu has gained lovely golden griddle marks.

03 In the meantime, in a bowl, whisk together the olive oil, lemon juice and mustard. Chop the herbs. Add these along with the garlic and seasoning and mix well.

04 When the tofu is ready, place it in a tray or large container and pour the marinade ensuring all slices are well coated. Leave in the fridge for a couple of hours or overnight if possible.

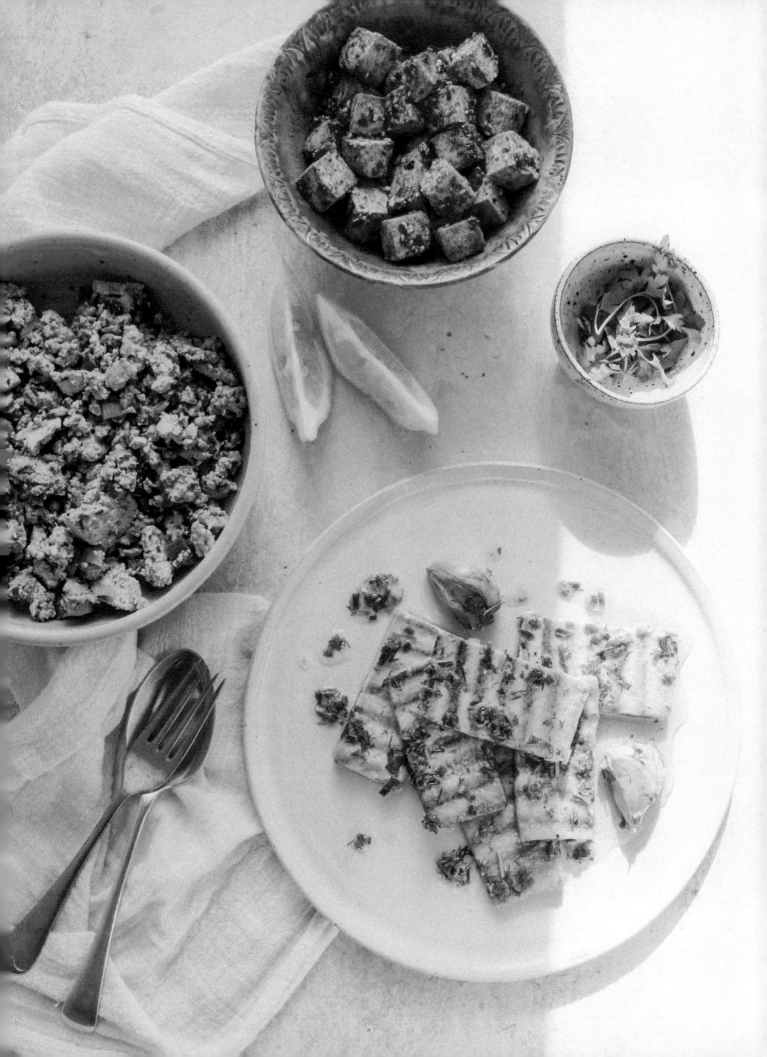

Harissa Tofu

Ingredients

- 300g super firm tofu (preferably organic)
- 1tbsp Harissa paste
- juice of 1/2 lemon
- 2tbsp olive oil
- salt and pepper, to taste
- 1tbsp sesame seeds

Prep: **10** min Cook: **20** min Servings: **4**

Directions

01 Pre-heat the oven to 200°C.

02 Drain the tofu block and dry it using a clean tea towel or kitchen paper to remove as much moisture as you can. Cut the tofu into bite-sized cubes.

03 In a bowl, mix together the Harissa, lemon juice, olive oil, salt and pepper. Toss the tofu in this marinade until all sides are covered.

04 Place the tofu in a roasting tray and roast for 20 minutes. Once baked, sprinkle with the sesame seeds and keep in an airtight container in the fridge.

Scrambled Tofu

Ingredients

- 300g firm tofu (preferably organic)
- 2tbsp olive oil
- 4 spring onions
- 1tbsp nutritional yeast
- 1tsp turmeric
- 1.5tsp garlic powder
- 1.5tbsp soy sauce
- 2tbsp almond or oat milk
- 1tbsp chopped chives
- salt and pepper, to taste

Prep: **10** min Cook: **10** min Servings: **4**

Directions

01 Heat the olive oil in a non-stick frying pan. Slice the spring onions finely and sauté in the olive oil for a few minutes.

02 To the spring onions, add the nutritional yeast, turmeric, garlic powder and soy sauce. Stir and cook for 1 minute.

03 Crumble the tofu into the pan and stir until the tofu is evenly coated. Cook for 3 to 5 minutes on medium heat.

04 Stir in the almond or oat milk and cook for another minute. Add the chives and season to taste.

No single number is a
complete picture of
your INDIVIDUAL
health

#manalivinghealing

Bacon Tempeh

Ingredients

Prep: **10** min (+ marinating)   Cook: **7** min   Servings: **4**

- 200g tempeh (preferably organic)
- 1tbsp olive oil
- 4tbsp reduced salt soy sauce
- 1tbsp rice wine vinegar
- 1tbsp maple syrup
- 1tsp smoked paprika
- 4 garlic cloves, bashed

Directions

01   Slice the tempeh longitudinally into 8 equal slices.

02   In a bowl, whisk all remaining ingredients (except the garlic cloves). Pour into a container big enough to store the tempeh slices in a way they are completely covered by the marinade. Add the tempeh and garlic cloves and keep in the fridge. It can be stored for 5 days and the flavours will develop more as it goes.

03   When you're ready to eat, sauté in a little olive oil on a non-stick frying pan until golden on both sides.

Note: This is one of my favourite ways to eat tempeh. It goes really well with a kale salad, chopped and tossed into pasta or with the Super Rice on page 34.

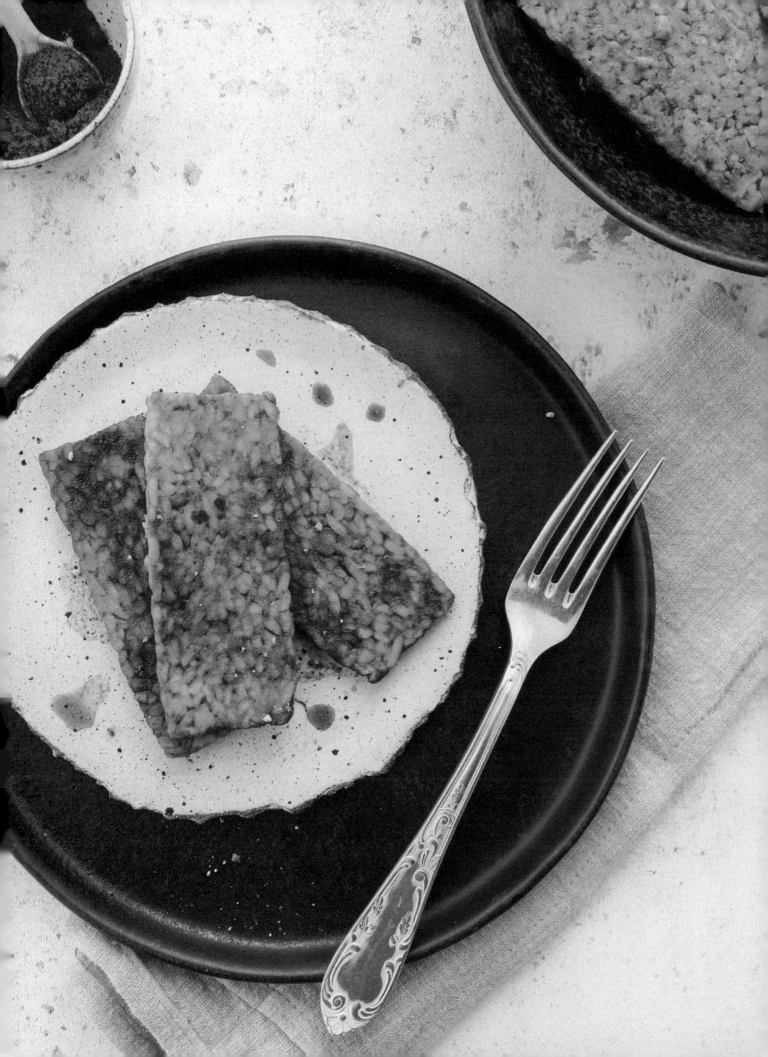

Roasted Butternut Squash

Ingredients

- 600g butternut squash
- 3tbsp olive oil
- 2 bay leaves
- 5 garlic cloves, bashed
- 1tsp chili flakes
- salt and pepper, to taste

Directions

01 Pre-heat the oven to 200°C. Peel, deseed and slice the butternut squash into 2cm slices.

02 Place the butternut squash slices in a roasting tray, drizzle with the olive oil, season with the chilli flakes, salt and pepper. Toss in the bay leaves and garlic.

03 Roast for 40 minutes or until is soft and caramelised on the edges.

Note: This is probably the simplest recipe in this book but no less delicious! My mother used to make this butternut squash side almost every week during the colder months and it still fills me with nostalgia whenever I eat it.

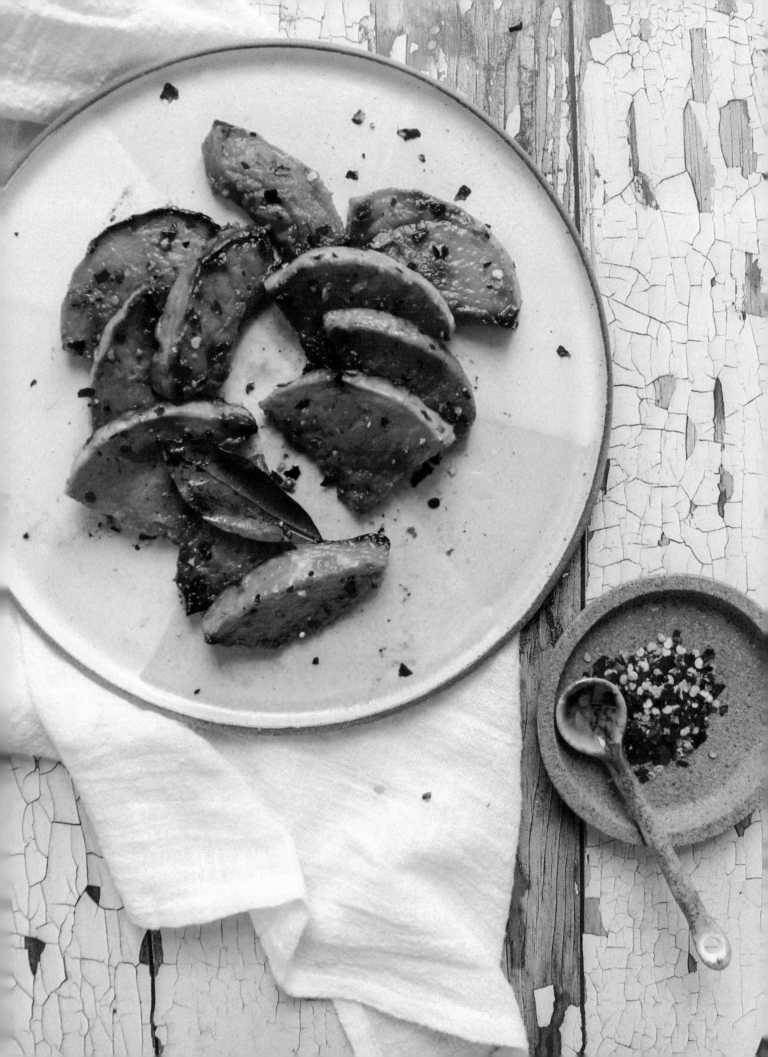

Simple Red Bean Salad

Ingredients

- 150g baby sweet peppers
- 2tbsp extra-virgin olive oil
- 200g cherry tomatoes
- 4 spring onions
- 20g coriander
- 1 can of red kidney beans
- 4 tbsp raw organic apple cider vinegar (or according to your taste)
- salt & pepper, to taste

Prep: **15** min Cook: **20** min Servings: **4**

Directions

01 Pre-heat the oven to 180ªC. Halve and deseed the peppers. Place in a roasting tray, season with salt and pepper and drizzle with 1tbsp olive oil. Roast for 20 minutes.

02 Quarter the cherry tomatoes, slice the spring onions and chop the coriander. Drain and rinse the kidney beans.

03 When the peppers are roasted, remove from the oven and chop into bite-sized pieces if needed. Combine all ingredients in a large bowl, including the remaining tablespoon of olive oil, and season to taste.

Note: This is one of my favourite recipes and is something I make every week. Equally delicious if you replace the kidney beans for sweetcorn.

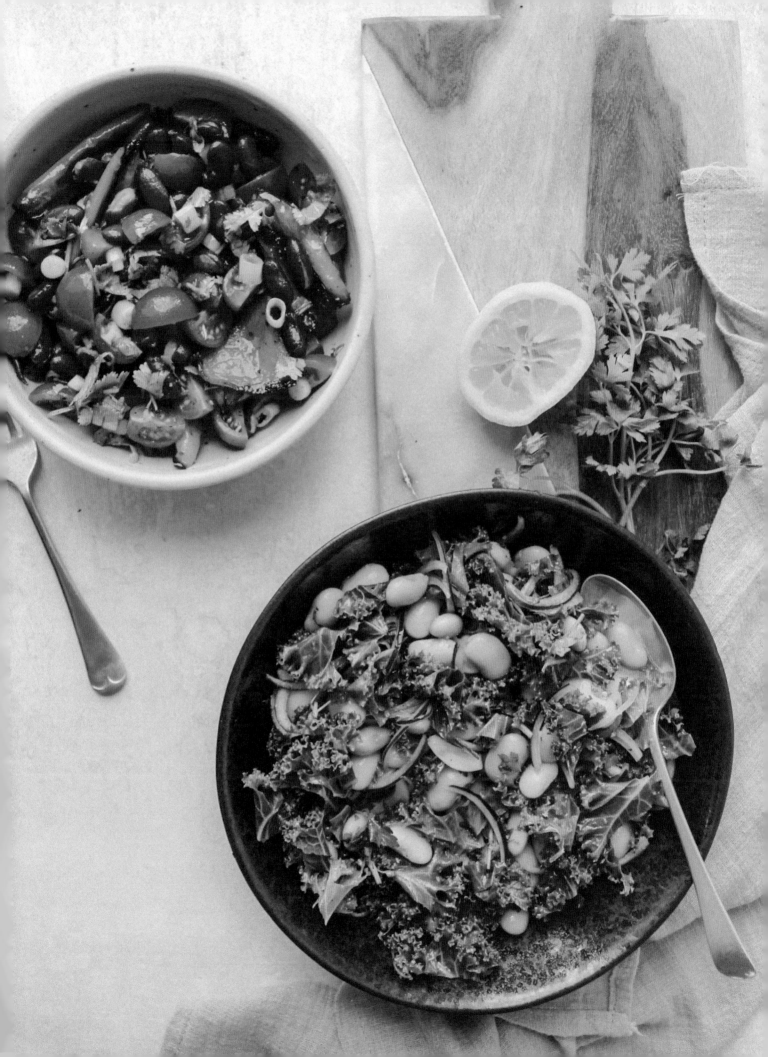

Lemony Butter Beans & Kale

Ingredients

Prep: **15** min   Cook: **5** min   Servings: **4**

- 100g kale
- 1 can of butter beans
- 1/4 red onion
- 10g parsley
- extra virgin olive oil
- juice and zest of 1/2 lemon
- salt and pepper

Directions

01 Steam or boil the kale for 5 minutes. Drain and rinse the beans. Finely slice the red onion and chop the parsley.

02 In a large bowl, combine the kale, beans, onion, parsley, lemon juice and zest. Season to taste.

03 Enjoy served warm or cold.

Note: Legumes like beans, chickpeas and lentils are not only a great source of plant protein, they have proven benefits when it comes to reducing the risk of stroke and some types of cancer.

"Be easy. Take your time. You are coming home to yourself."

- *Nayyirah Waheed*

Simple Garlic & Chili Greens

Ingredients

- 200g tenderstem broccoli
- 200g green beans
- 1 small garlic clove, grated
- 2tbsp olive oil
- 2tbsp raw apple cider vinegar
- 1 small chilli, sliced
- 1tbsp sesame seeds
- salt & pepper

Prep: **10** m Cook: **5** m Servings: **6**

Directions

01 Bring a kettle to boil. To a large pan, add the broccoli and green beans and add the water to cover. Add a pinch of salt and cook for 5 minutes. You can also steam if you prefer.

02 Grate the garlic. To a small bowl add the garlic, olive oil and apple cider vinegar. Whisk together.

03 When the greens are cooked, drain* and add to a food container or salad bow. Add the dressing and mix well. Top with the sliced chillies and sesame seeds.

Note: You can use any greens here, such as kale and spring greens for example. Having a big batch of cooked greens in the fridge is a great way of complementing any meal and boosting your antioxidant intake.

*If you're making the Warm Spring Salad (page 54) on the same day, reserve the cooking water and use it to boil the peas. This will not only keep the nutrients in the water, but also reduce washing up.

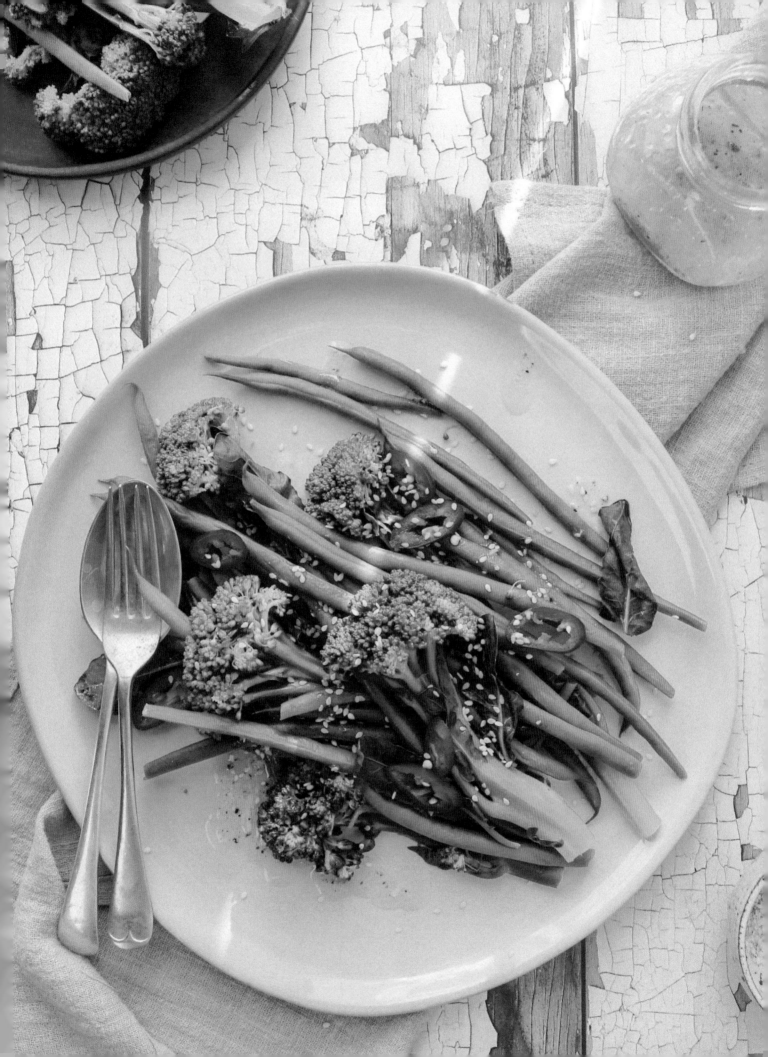

Spicy Sweet Potatoes

Ingredients

Prep: **10** m   Cook: **35** m   Servings: **6**

- 4 medium sweet potatoes, scrubbed
- 2tsp smoked paprika
- 1tsp garlic powder
- 1tsp oregano
- 1/2tsp chilli powder (optional)
- 2tbsp olive oil
- salt and pepper

Directions

01 Pre-heat the oven to 200°C (fan). Cut the sweet potatoes into 1cm fingers.

02 To a roasting tray add the sweet potatoes and all other ingredients. Mix well until the sweet potatoes are evenly coated in seasoning.

03 Roast for 35 minutes or until the sweet potato is cooked and slightly charred on the edges.

Note: Sweet potatoes are a great source of vitamins and antioxidants and taste delicious with any of the meal prep recipes in this book.

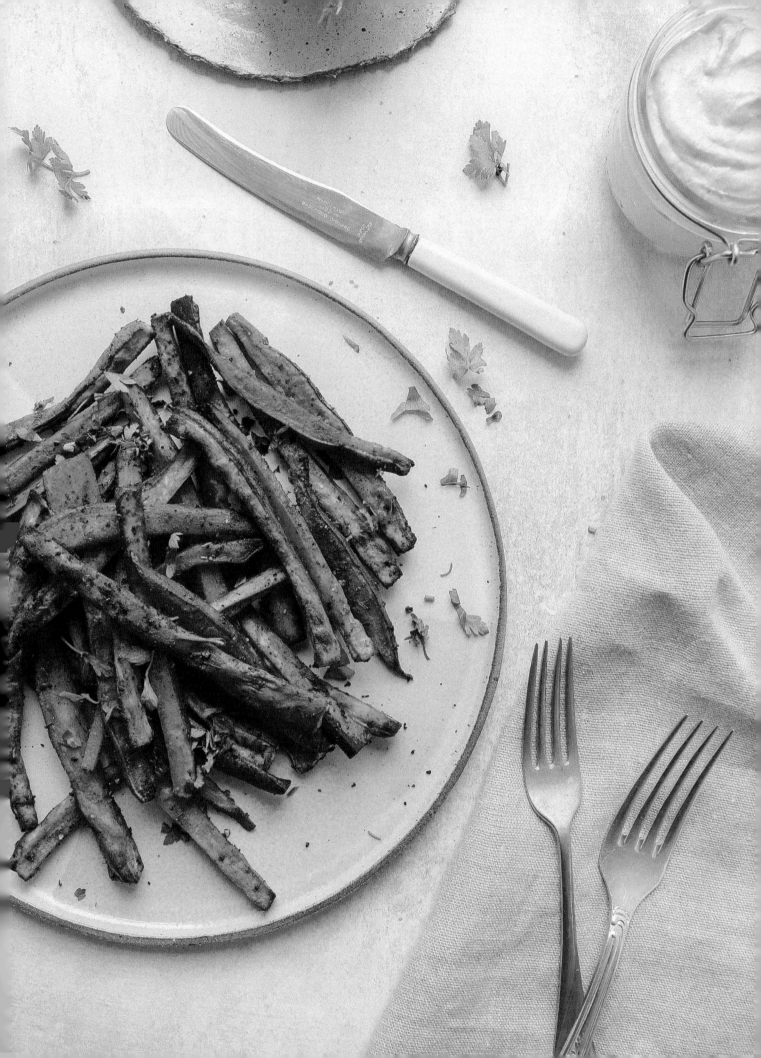

Warm Spring Salad

Ingredients

Prep: **10** m   Cook: **8** m   Servings: **6**

- 150g frozen peas
- 200g curly kale, stalks removed and leaves roughly chopped
- 120g mangetout
- 100g radishes
- 15g mint, leaves only
- salt & pepper

Directions

01   Boil a kettle. To a tall pan, add the frozen peas and boil for 8 minutes. Five minutes before the end, place a steamer on top of the pan to steam cook the kale and mangetout.

02   Thinly slice the radishes. Once the veg are cooked, stir them into the bowl with the dressing and add the radishes and mint leaves.

03   Serve with the Maple & Mustard Dressing on page 58.

Note: I love this salad served with some hummus and the sweet potatoes on page 52.

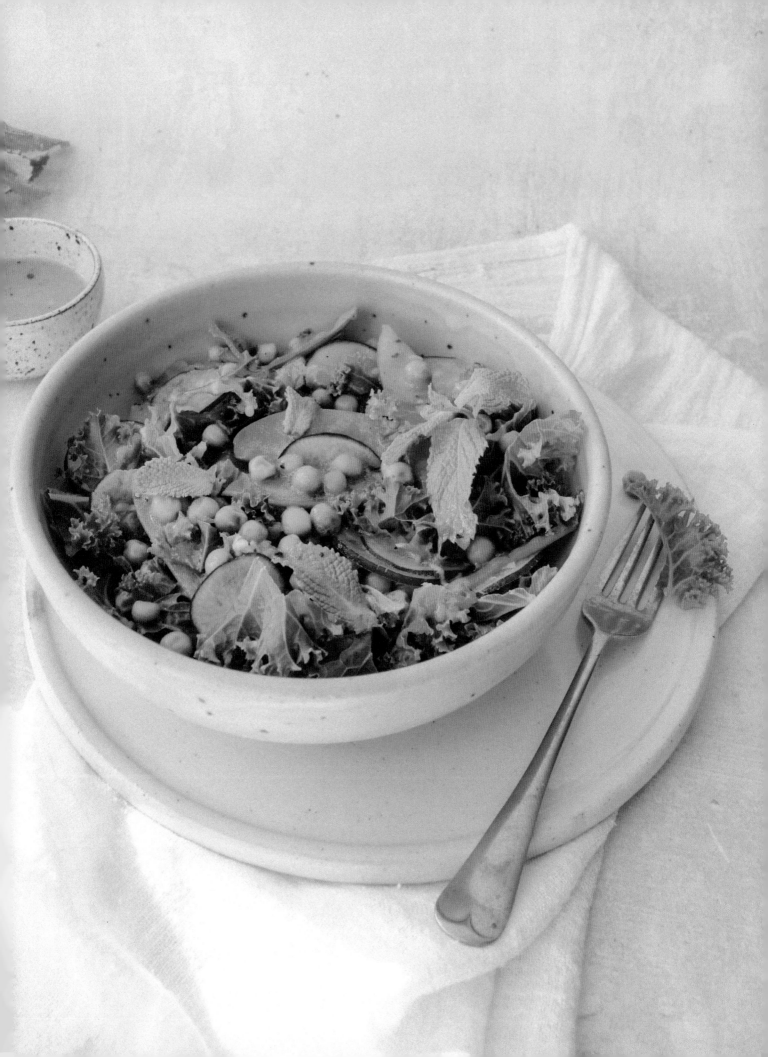

Pulled Mushrooms

Ingredients

- 1 small red onion
- 1tbsp olive oil
- 250g king oyster mushrooms
- 1tsp smoked paprika
- 1tsp garlic powder
- 1/2tsp cumin
- 1/2tsp chipotle chili powder
- salt & pepper

Prep: **10** m   Cook: **15** m   Servings: **4** m

Directions

01 Finely dice the red onion. In a frying pan, heat up the olive oil and fry the onion on medium-low heat until translucent.

02 Cut the tops off the mushrooms and finely slice. Using a fork, shred the mushroom stalks.

03 Add the spices to the onions (except the salt) and fry for a minute.

Turn the heat up and add the pulled mushrooms to the pan. Leave to cook undisturbed for a couple of minutes. Stir and cook undisturbed, again, until they look brown all over. Season with salt.

Note: Delicious served over wholewheat tortillas, with chopped cucumber, spring onion and avocado slices.

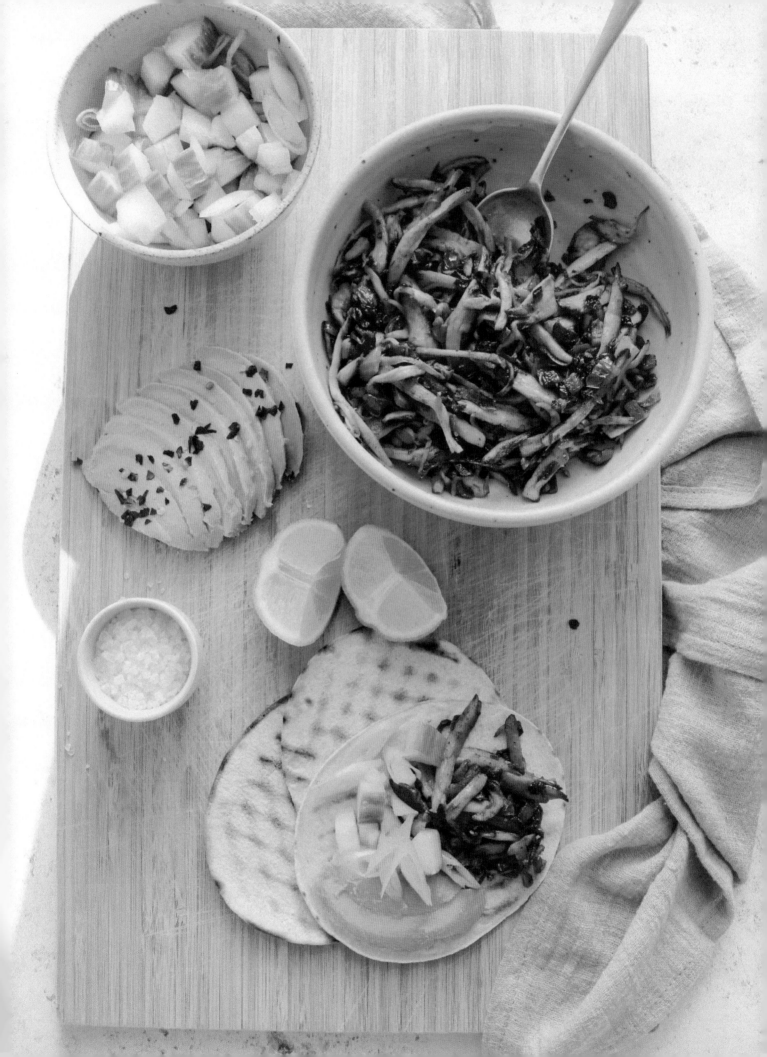

Maple & Mustard Dressing

Ingredients

- 4tbsp olive oil
- 4tbsp raw apple cider vinegar
- 1tbsp wholegrain mustard
- 1/2tbsp Dijon mustard
- 1tsp oregano
- salt and pepper, to taste

Prep: **5** min Servings: **makes 150 ml**

Directions

01 Whisk all ingredients together in a medium bowl. Store in an airtight container in the fridge.

Herby Yoghurt Dressing

Ingredients

- 200g oat yoghurt
- 1tbsp olive oil
- juice of 1/2 lemon
- 1tsp garlic powder
- 5g dill
- 10g chives
- 10g flat leaf parsley
- salt and pepper, to taste

Prep: **5** min Servings: **makes 250ml**

Directions

01 Add all ingredients to a food processor and blend well until you have a creamy dressing.

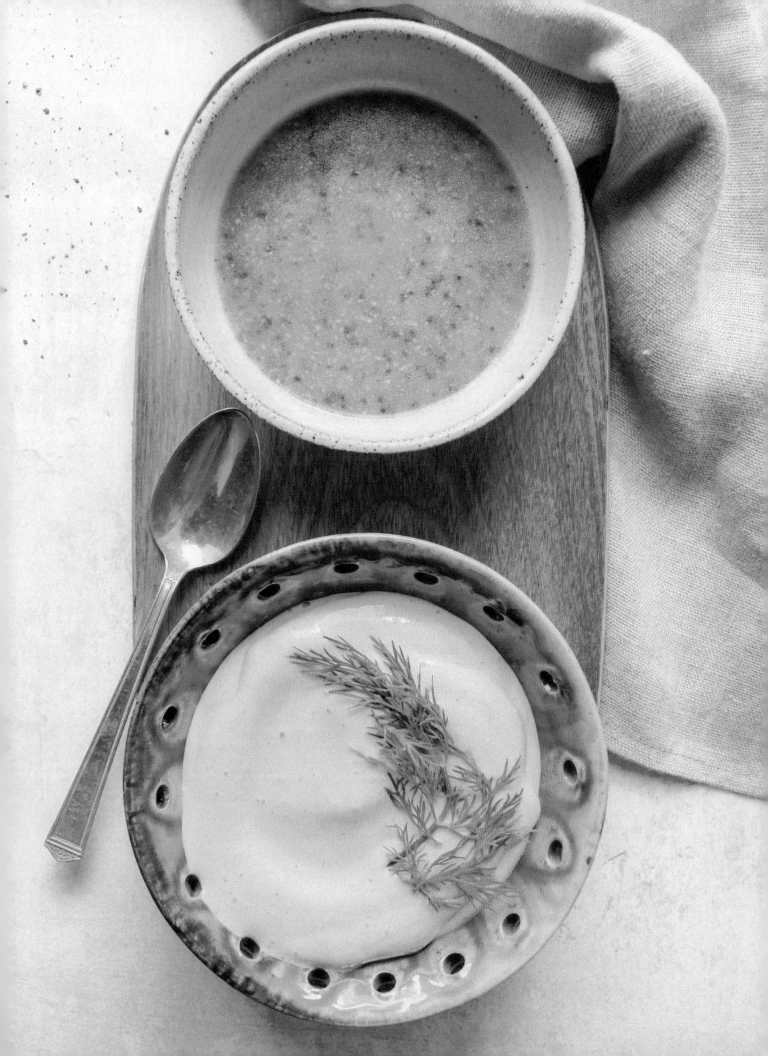

"We are one integrated being. We need to take care of all aspects of ourselves."

- Mark Hyman

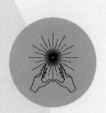

Sweets

Choccy-Nana Loaf

A cross between a banana bread and a brownie, this is a firm favourite in our house.

Ingredients

Prep: **15** min   Cook: **60** min   Servings: **12**

- 200g coconut sugar
- 4tbsp cacao powder (not cocoa)
- 120g brown rice flour
- 70g almond flour
- 1tsp bicarbonate of soda
- 1tsp baking powder
- 4 very ripe bananas, mashed with a fork (optional: + 1 extra banana for decoration)
- 50g coconut oil, melted
- 200ml almond milk
- 1/2 vanilla pod, seeds scraped
- 50g cacao nibs

Directions

01 Pre-heat your oven to 180° (fan). Line a loaf tin with baking paper.

02 In a large bowl combine all dry ingredients: coconut sugar, cacao, brown rice and almond flour, baking soda and baking powder. Mix well to combine and get rid of any clumps.

03 In a separate bowl, combine the mashed bananas, coconut oil, almond milk and vanilla.

04 Gradually, stir the dry ingredients in, mixing well as you go and until everything is combined. Fold in most of the cacao nibs (you can leave a few behind to sprinkle on top).

05 Pour the cake mixture into the prepared tin. Top with the remaining cacao nibs and banana and bake for 60 minutes - do a check at 45 minutes so you can adjust the baking time depending on your oven. You might need to cover loosely with foil if it starts to look too dark on top.

06 Let it cool in the tin and transfer to a rack to cool completely before slicing with a serrated knife. It's even fudgier when stored in the fridge in an airtight container.

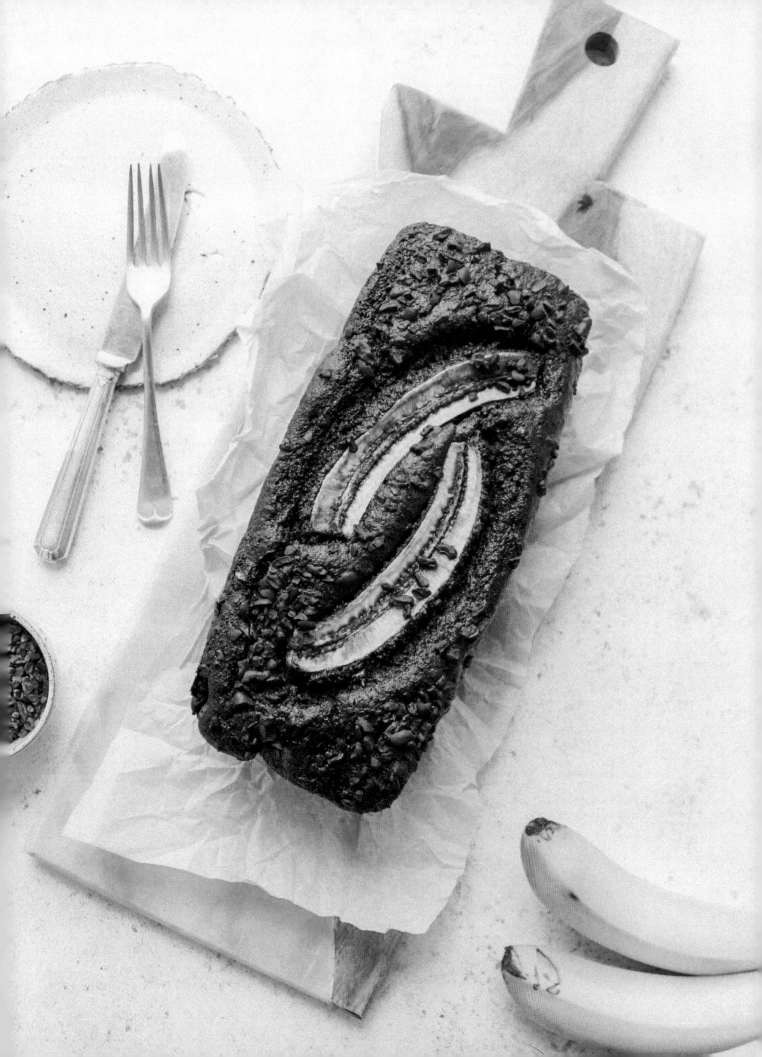

Mini Key Lime Pies

Ingredients

Prep: **30** m + soaking and chilling   Servings: **9**

For the base

- 3/4 cup chopped dates
- 1 + 1/4 cups ground almonds
- 1 tbsp coconut oil, melted

For the filling

- 1 + 1/2 cups cashew nuts soaked overnight in the fridge or for 1h in very hot water
- 1 tsp vanilla extract
- juice of 2 limes
- zest of 3 limes
- 1/4 cup brown rice milk
- 1/4 cup coconut oil, melted
- 1/2 cup agave syrup
- 200g thick coconut yoghurt

Note: these mini pies are equally light and indulgent. The creamy filling is made with cashews which are rich in heart-loving fats, zinc and magnesium.

Directions

01 Line a muffin tray with muffin cases.

02 To make the base, blitz the dates, almond flour and coconut oil in a food processor until you have a paste you can form. If this is difficult, add a tbsp of water but be careful adding more as you want a dough-like consistency.

03 Divide the mixture for the 9 muffin cases, pressing down with the back of a spoon or your thumb until it evenly covers the bottom. Put in the fridge while you continue.

04 For the filling, add all ingredients to your food processor and blend until you have a creamy mixture (it can take 2 minutes or so until it all comes together).

05 Divide equally amongst the prepared tins and pop in the freezer for a couple of hours or overnight. Remove from the freezer 15 minutes before serving and top with a dollop of coconut yoghurt.

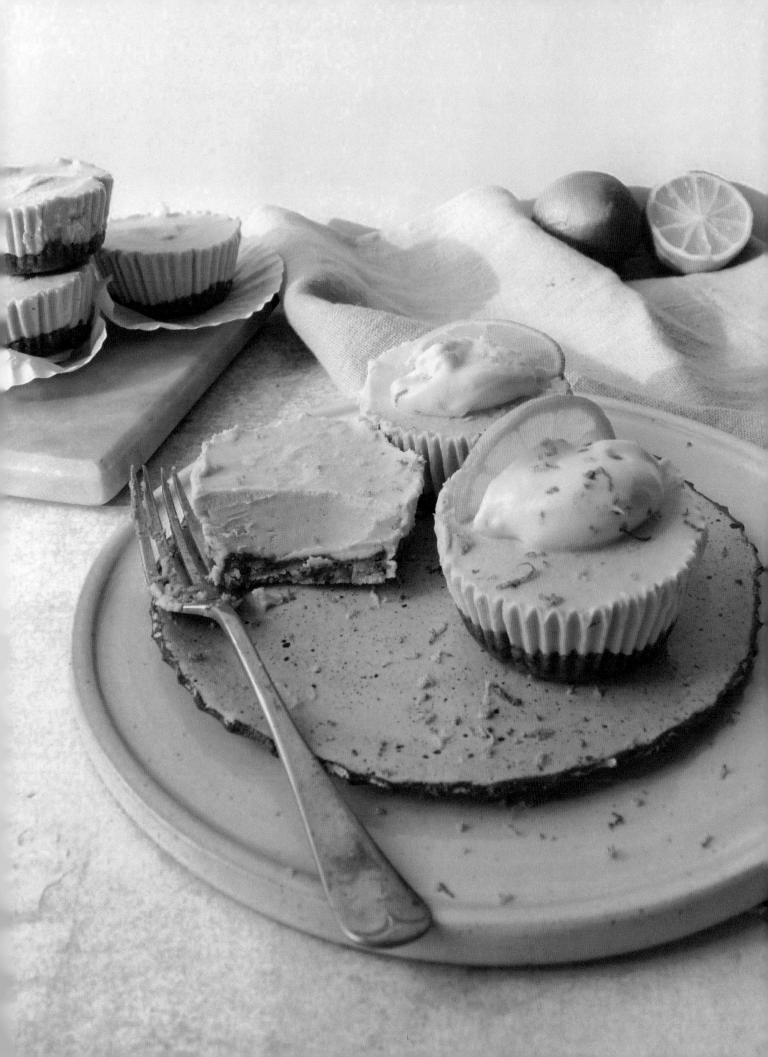

Coconut Macaroons

Ingredients

Prep: **10** m   Cook: **35** m   Servings: **10**

- 2 cups desiccated coconut
- 1/2 cup ground almonds
- 1/4 cup chia seeds
- 2tbsp coconut oil
- 1 vanilla pod, seeds removed
- 1 cup coconut milk
- 1/4 cup maple cyrup
- a pinch of salt

Directions

01 Pre-heat your oven to 170°C fan. Line a baking sheet with greaseproof paper.

02 In a medium saucepan, melt the coconut oil on a low heat. Add all other ingredients and cook for 5 minutes until you have a creamy mixture.

03 Place half of the mixture in a food processor and blend well. Mix in the rest of the desiccated coconut.

04 Scoop tablespoons of the mixture and roll into uniform balls. Place in the lined baking sheet and bake for 30 minutes or until golden.

Note: These macaroons are great as they are, but if you want to elevate them, dip in melted chocolate and set in the fridge.

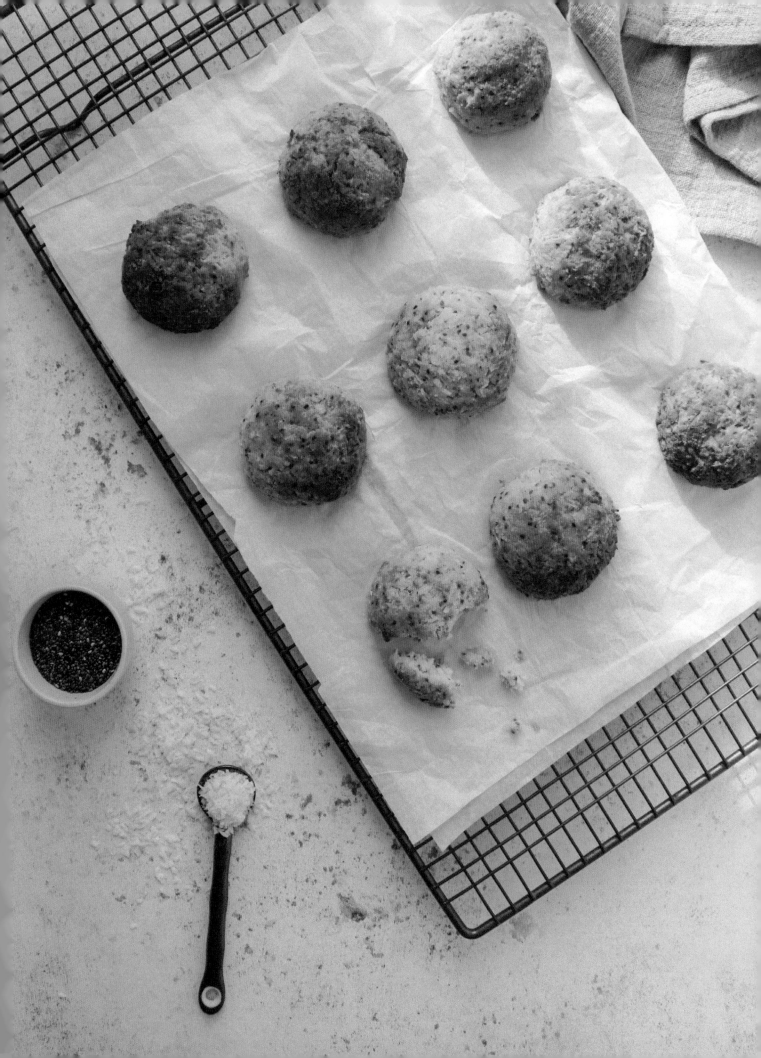

Probiotic Chocolate Mousse

Ingredients

- 1 cup blanched hazelnuts, soaked overnight or for 1h in hot water
- 1 cup vanilla flavoured coconut yogurt, made with live cultures
- 4tbsp maple syrup
- 1tbsp cacao powder

Directions

01   Drain the hazelnuts. Add all ingredients to a blender and blend well until you have a creamy mixture.

02   Divide equally amongst 3 ramekins and chill in the fridge overnight.

Note: Whilst traditional chocolate mousse is heavy in refined sugar, this recipe is incredibly well balanced due to the the tangy yoghurt and the slight bitterness of the raw cacao.

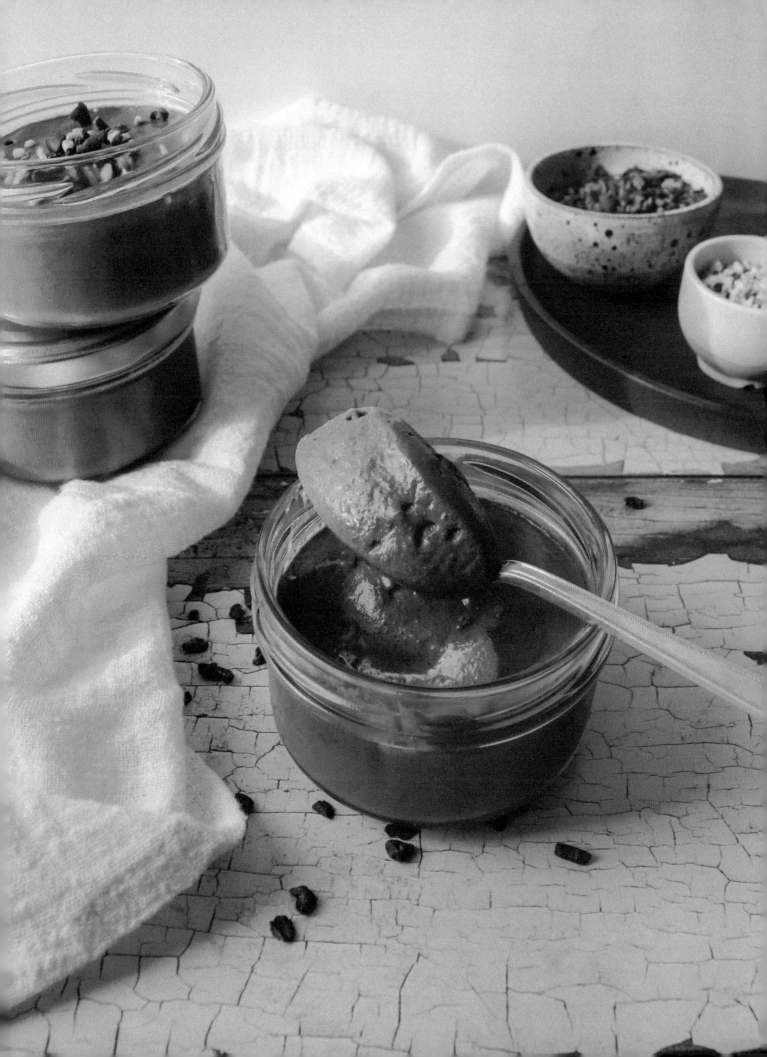

Move Well

Improve Your Energy and Feel Stronger

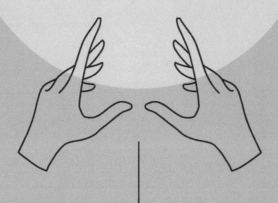

Move Well

According to the UK's National Health Service exercise guidelines, we should aim to do at least 150 minutes of moderate intensity (or 75 minutes of vigorous intensity) activity a week, including strengthening activities at least 2 days a week (10).

This is only about 20 minutes a day but, according to Public Health England, 34% of men and 42% of women are not active enough (11).

This contributes to 1 in every 6 deaths in the UK and represents a major burden to the healthcare system (12).

We know the benefits of exercise but still find it difficult to show up for ourselves.

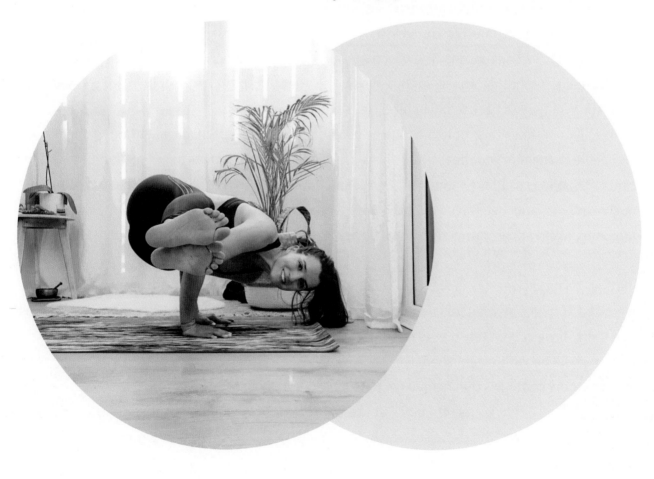

Move Well

So why exactly should we exercise?

We all know that exercise helps us maintain a healthy weight (13) but the benefits go way beyond that. Consistent physical activity also improves ageing (14), increases our resting metabolic rate (15), decreases incidence of chronic disease (16), improves sleep quality (17), increases oxygen capacity, bone density (especially for weight based exercises), raises good cholesterol, lowers blood pressure and reduces the incidence of cardiovascular disease by 45% (16)!

As if this wasn't enough, 150 minutes a week of moderate physical activity has shown a 20% reduced risk of breast cancer in women, as well as better recovery outcomes for those affected (18).

Why is it difficult to maintain a consistent workout routine?

From my experience, one reason why making exercising a habit is so difficult is because we workout for the wrong reasons. The vast majority of women I coach exercise to lose weight. They start running or hitting the gym but when this doesn't produce visible results, they lose motivation and revert back to old habits.

No one likes to hear this, but to achieve sustainable outcomes, it will take time until you see noticeable changes in your health and appearance. You cannot stop because you don't see instant results. Usually it will take months, if not years, until you're able to look back and realise how much stronger and healthier you feel. So you need to exercise for all the wonderful health outcomes listed above, rather than the weight loss or the six pack.

Another common reason is lack of willpower or motivation. In my opinion, motivation is overrated. It might be what you need to take the first step but motivation will not keep you going long term. If we cannot rely on the reminder that prompts us to initiate a habit, then it is unlikely that habit will become established.

Here are some strategies that helped me to establish a consistent workout routine:

1. Schedule your workouts (4) - block at least four periods of 45 minutes in your calendar each week. Write down the exercises you'll do or links to online videos, so when you're ready to workout you know exactly what to do.

2. Let go of perfectionism - I cannot say I give 100% at every single workout but I show up for

Move Well

myself EVERY SINGLE TIME. Some days you'll be tired or not "in the mood" but do not let this stop you. More often than not you'll still have a great workout once you start and if not, do what you can without judgements. This will build your consistency.

3. <u>Surround yourself with active people</u> (4) - for better or worse, other people's habits rub off on us. For example, if you want to take up wild swimming, look for local groups to connect with people who have shared interests. Bonus points as they will keep you accountable too!

I'm sold, where do I start?

Make it yours! You know yourself better than anyone else so think about what you love to do. One thing I learned is that I need variety, so I never repeat a workout. The key is to find different things to keep you fit, explore the exercises that feel like play rather than a chore. Try different gym classes, experiment with running, biking, hiking or dancing. A great playlist can also make a huge difference when it comes to making a workout more fun.

My personal weekly workout plan includes; five days of strength training (19) (upper body, lower body and three full body), two yoga classes and one rest day. For this programme, try and incorporate five workouts a week. Ideally these would be 45 minutes each, but if this is too much, start with 30 minutes or even 20. The key here is to move consistently.

I'm not a personal trainer, but there are some great free resources out there which can help you with building a workout routine. Keep it simple! You'll be surprised at how effective walking and simple strength exercises can be.

Here are some of my favourite free resources to get you started:

Yoga for Beginners: *Yoga with Adriene*

Yoga: *Cat Meffan*, *Alo Yoga*

Fitness and Yoga: *Alo Moves*, *Yoga by Candace*

Workouts: *Lilly Sabri*, *SWEAT*, *Heather Robertson*, *p.volve*

Dance Workouts: *305 Fitness*

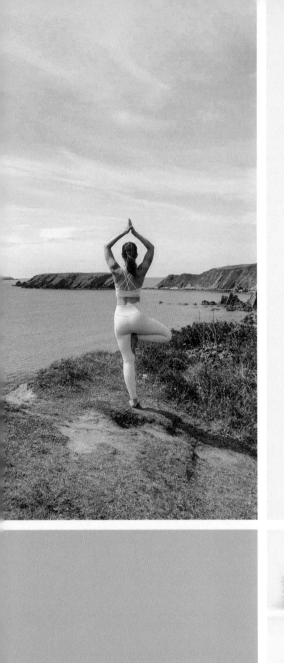
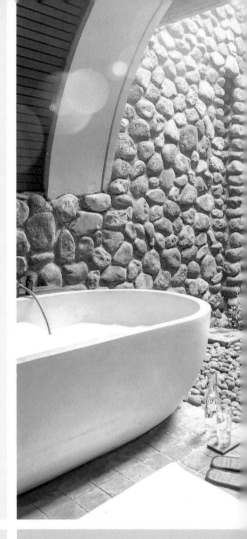
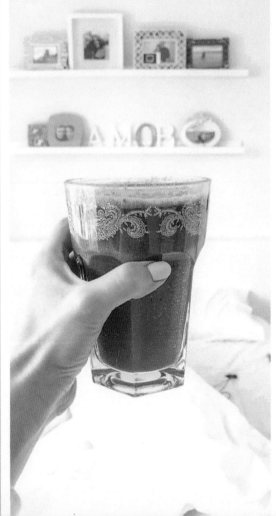

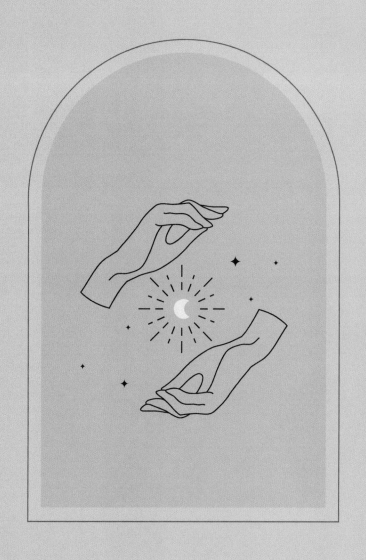

Sleep Well

Let Your Body Recover

Sleep Well

Sleep not only impacts your energy levels, but is an essential part of our recovery, memory consolidation and cognitive function (20).

Lack of sleep and/or poor quality sleep de-regulates our hormones which negatively impacts our metabolism, appetite and mood (20). It has also been linked to decreased immunity, early mortality and increased ageing, as well as increased risk of certain chronic diseases e.g. obesity, type 2 diabetes, high blood pressure and Alzheimer's (21).

Long gone are the days of "I'll sleep when I'm dead".

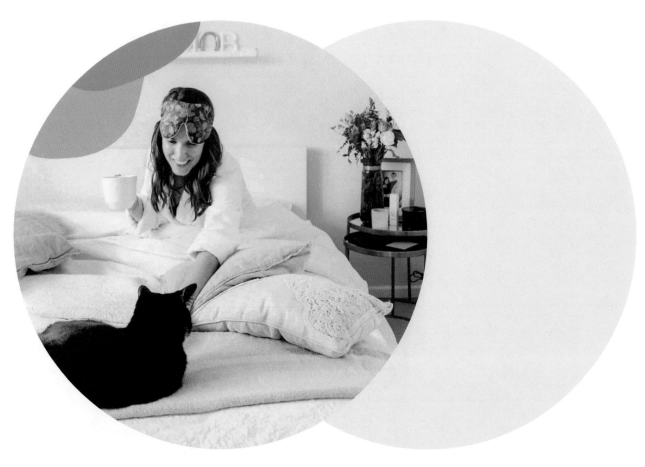

Knowing how essential sleep is, you'd think we would prioritise this area of wellness. However, a report published by the the UK's Sleep Council shows that the average adult only gets 6 hours and 35 minutes of sleep per night (22) - significantly under the 7 - 9 hours recommended by the Sleep Foundation (23).

Sleep deprivation costs the UK 's economy over £40 billion a year (24), yet there is a lack of education on the importance of sleep. So, let's start with a brief summary of how sleep works.

Thanks to our natural circadian rhythm, most people feel sleepy between 22:00 and 23:00 (25). Once asleep, you will go through different sleep stages which combined, form a cycle (see page 78 for more information). So it's essential that you determine YOUR ideal bedtime and stick with it.

One aspect I love about setting a regular bedtime is the possibility of creating a mindful bedtime routine. Spending 30 minutes winding down before bed will help you to feel more relaxed and fall asleep quicker.

Your bedtime routine should suit your lifestyle and bioindividuality, but here are some of my favourite suggestions:

Everything you do, you do BETTER with a good night of sleep

- having a bath or giving yourself a facial massage
- meditate or quiet reflection for 10 minutes to clear your mind
- experiment with essential oils such as lavender, vanilla, ylang ylang or jasmine

Because everything in our body is connected, there are a number of factors which affect our sleep. We know that sleep impacts our appetite, however, our diet also impacts sleep.

A diverse diet, rich in essential vitamins and minerals plus adequate hydration are the foundation for a good night of sleep. For example, B vitamins are directly related to sleep regulation (26).

Also, as caffeine has a half-life of 3 - 5 hours (27), you should avoid it at least 8 hours before going to bed. Therefore, improved sleep is another benefit you can gain from following the nutritious recipes in this book.

Vitamin D also has a major impact on sleep regulation. Vitamin D is produced by our bodies in the presence of sunlight and helps keep our biological clocks in tune, so getting even 15 minutes of natural morning light will also aid the sleep process (28).

If you live in a northern latitude country, you may consider taking a Vitamin D3 (5000IU) supplement, but always speak with your healthcare professional beforehand as they can interact with other medicines or supplements.

There is also mounting evidence surrounding the positive effect of regular exercise in relation to sleep quality and duration. Exercising can help you fall asleep quicker and it has also been associated with better quality of sleep in those who exercise three or more days a week (29). Exercise can also have an indirect benefit on sleep by both reducing stress levels and supporting weight maintenance. This means reduced likelihood of lying awake at night and improvements on the severity of obstructive sleep apnea for those affected (30).

We could not talk about sleep optimisation without discussing the influence of our environment in promoting a good night of sleep (31):

- Light - This has a profound effect on sleep since exposure to light, more especially blue light from electronic devices, turns off melatonin production making it more difficult to fall asleep.
- Sound - This can be a major sleep disruptor for some people. So, if you struggle to fall asleep or wake up during the night because of noise, consider using earplugs or a sound machine. Also, soothing sounds might help you relax and drift into sleep more easily.
- Temperature - Your body temperature naturally drops off in the evening to stimulate melatonin production. Research suggests that an ideal bedroom temperature is between 16°C - 18°C. Check if your mattress has a summer and winter side and turn it according to the season. Good quality bedsheets and an appropriate duvet for the time of the year can also help in regulating the temperature when you sleep.

Stages of the Sleep Cycle

On average, each cycle lasts for about 90 minutes and ideally occurs 4 - 6 times a night (25).

Stage 1

Very light sleep, makes up about 5% of your total sleep time.

Stage 2

Deeper sleep state, this is where the brain produces rhythmic brain waves and represents about 50% of your sleep.

Stage 3

The deep or delta sleep, the most restorative stage of sleep where the body repairs and the immune system is strengthened.

REM (rapid eye movement)

The mental restoration and memory consolidation stage. The time between each REM cycle represents the length of each cycle.

Top Tips

01
Audit Your Bedroom
Use blackout blinds or an eye mask, soft sheets etc. to create the perfect environment

02
Set A Bedtime Alarm
Ensures consistency and gives you time to wind down

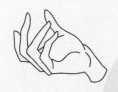

03
Have A Bath
Use magnesium salts for extra relaxation - bonus points for candlelight

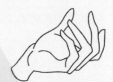

04
Avoid Screens
No TV or electronic device use after 9pm

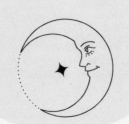

05
Meditate
Even 10 minutes helps to clear the mind

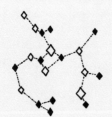

06
Go Outside
Be exposed to natural light early in the day

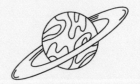

When you let go of old habits, you create space for something better.

#manalivinghealing

The Programme

Time To Put Your Learning Into Practice

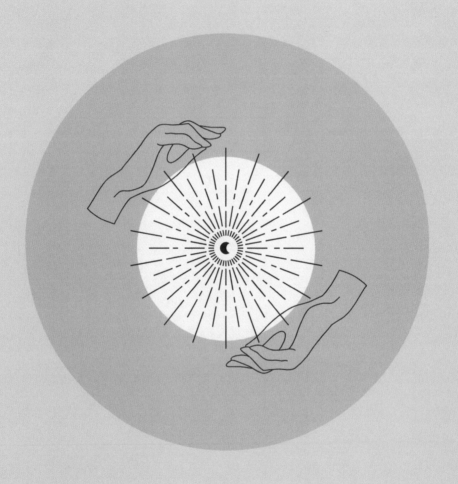

The Programme

If you've got this far, you'll have realised that there are no quick fixes when it comes to your wellness. You have to put in the work, but I promise you it will be worth it! Whether you start this programme or not, the next 30 days will pass regardless - so it's up to you how you use them.

If you've skipped to this chapter go back and read the previous ones, as understanding the reasons behind the programme is an important part of sticking with it for the next 30 days and beyond.

A lot of programmes will suggest you change one thing at a time within your life, but not this one.

Don't get me wrong, I still believe that implementing small, sustainable changes which build on each other is the best way to achieve long-lasting habit change.

However, these 3 pillars of wellness are so entwined, that you'll find more motivation and better results if you work on your diet, exercise and sleep together.

My hope is that, when the 30 days end, you won't notice because these habits will be so well ingrained, they won't feel like a programme or challenge anymore. Perhaps after 30 days you don't feel quite there yet, that's fine, take your time and continue the programme until you feel your habits are well established.

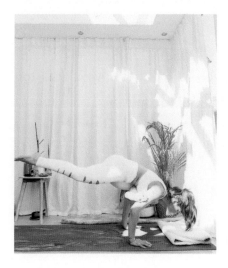
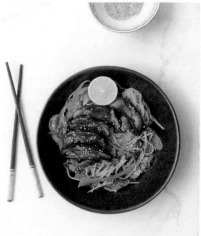
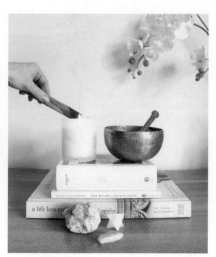

Before You Start

Your success will depend more on your planning than your motivation.

This is why I want you to get organised before the 30-days timeline actually begins. On the days before you're ready to start, take time to go through the actions on the next page. This will ensure you set yourself up for success and become familiar with planning your wellness routine.

Every Sunday (if you work a regular week), before you plan the week ahead, take some time to reflect on how the previous week went and if you need to make any changes to your routine. Also use this time to consider obstacles, anticipating times which may test you and plan for this. It'll be an exercise at first but, as you immerse yourself in the Mana Living Mindset, the appropriate choices for you (whether it's a slice of cake or a plate of broccoli) will come naturally and intuitively.

This programme won't last forever so as much as you can, try to stick with your meal prep, exercise, good sleep routine and proper hydration whilst reducing sugar, processed food and alcohol consumption.

This will help with kickstarting new habits by creating space for all the goodness that will come into your life.

After the programme ends you should have established a new lifestyle, so having a slice of pizza on a Friday night won't be a failure - it's all part of a balanced lifestyle.

However, it's important that after special days or holidays you go straight back to the habits you created. There is no space for an all-or-nothing mentality in this new lifestyle. Balance doesn't mean living perfectly 100% of the time, it means that you always go back to healthy rituals after a challenging day (or days).

Action Plan

Using all you've learnt so far, complete the actions below before starting your programme.

Eat Well

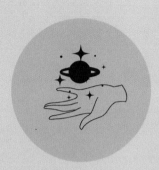

- Plan which meals from this book (or other sources) you'll be preparing
- Write a shopping list and buy all the ingredients you need
- Block some time on the days before starting the programme to meal prep and plan the order in which you'll be cooking everything to maximise your time
- Clean your pantry of anything that won't be serving you during this programme

Move Well

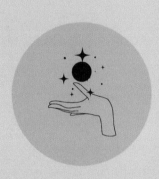

- Review your schedule and decide on the best time to workout each day
- Reserve 45 minute slots 5 days a week
- Book classes if you need to or choose the exact workouts you'll be doing each day and make a note of these
- If you are going to workout at home, order any equipment you might need (I use a set of adjustable weights and resistance bands)
- Initially, it might be worth having a full length mirror or your laptop/phone camera set up (even without recording) so you can check your form

Sleep Well

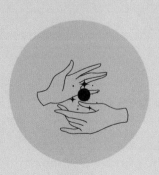

- Design your perfect bedtime routine and time it
- Set up a bedtime alarm, taking into consideration your bedtime routine and the amount of sleep you need
- Audit your bedroom and make sure everything is optimised for the perfect night of sleep

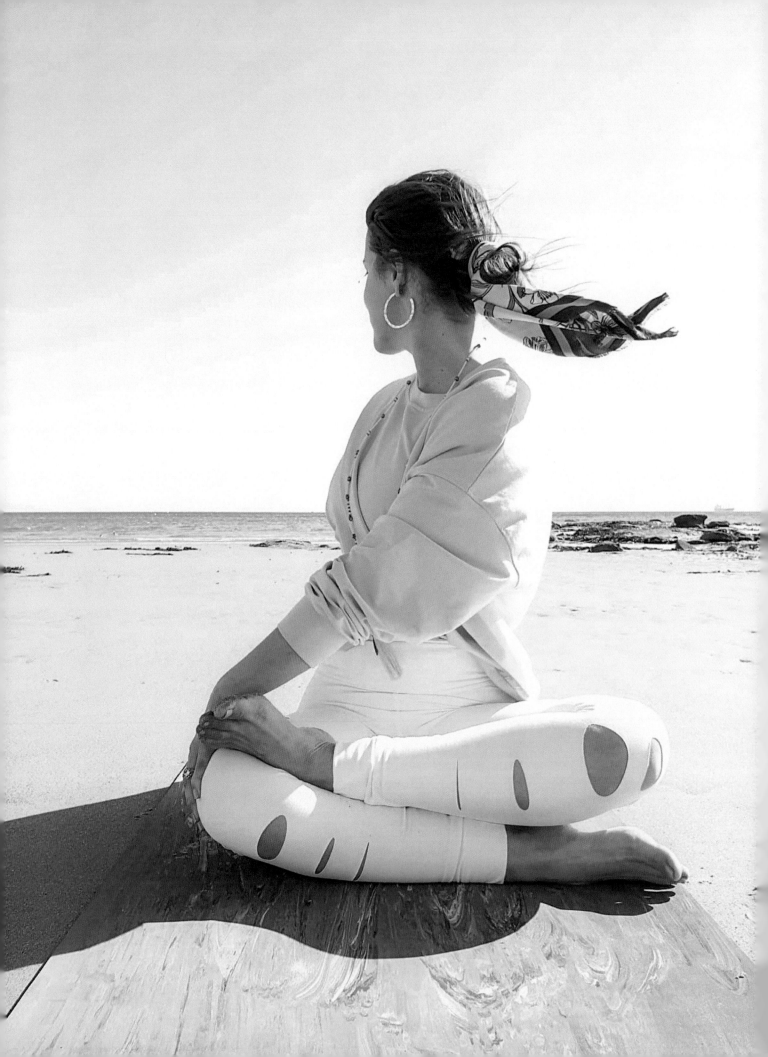

This Is Where The Magic Starts

Only 30 days to reset your lifestyle and transform your life. Make it count!

I have said this before and will say it again, commit to these 30 days to change your current habits and build a new lifestyle. You won't have to do it so strictly forever but you need to allow your body and mind time to adapt and optimise your new routine.

We'll be using the strategy of crowding out as much as possible. By filling your plate with veggies, you're crowding out unhealthy food. By filling some of your free time with exercise, you're crowding out habits that no longer serve you.

Over the next pages you'll find all the trackers and plans you need to monitor your progress and keep yourself accountable. Feel free to use them all or select the ones that fit your habit change strategy.

If you need external accountability, make sure to join our Facebook group (more information on page 89).

To keep you on track and motivated, there is a "30 Day Action Plan" on page 90. These are not replacements for your meal prep, exercise and sleep routine but rather suggestions to optimise your programme.

We tend to overestimate the good things we do and underestimate the less positive ones (e.g. we order a take away more often than we think we do). If the strategy of monitoring resonates with you, you'll love the daily habit trackers on pages 91 - 94.

The weekly planners on pages 95 and 96 are perfect for scheduling and makes building your new habits as convenient and easy and possible. Looking at your weekly schedule, use it to block out time for meal prepping and planning time for moving your body. Write down your exercise plan for each day, including the exact exercises or classes you'll do.

Finally, on page 97 you'll find the "Check-In With Yourself" assessment. Complete it on days 15 and 30 of the programme to assess your progress with each pillar we're working on. Compare it with the same parameters on the "Circle of Life" (page 9) you completed earlier.

Continue to build awareness and recognise how you're feeling with the lifestyle changes you've made. As you move forward, you'll become more connected to your intuition and will naturally select the choices which make you happiest.

Some days doing two yoga classes in a row will make you feel amazing, whereas others, your joy will come from a bowl of pasta curled up in front of the fire. Both have a place in a balanced lifestyle and it's your mindful awareness that will guide you. It will help you through days in which you believe you're too tired to workout (when you're actually being lazy).

It will stop you reaching for that processed dessert you don't enjoy that much, but you choose because you're emotional or bored.

When you opt for that dessert or bowl of chips there's no guilt attached to it because you choose it in full awareness of what your body and soul needs. Then when you return to your meal prep and exercise the day after, it's not to punish yourself, you're simply returning to your normal routine.

No cheat days, no diet culture, no calorie counting, no point system, no all-or-nothing mentality.

This is not a health kick, this is a transformational programme to support you in changing your habits and connecting to your needs and desires. To help you find freedom in your choices whilst feeling good about yourself.

You now know the importance that diet, exercise and sleep play in your life and wellbeing, you've learned about habit change strategies and have all the supportive trackers you need.

This is the first step towards an empowered way of living, with a sense of balance and control over your choices. Increased vitality, a new mindset and healthier way of life awaits you.

Join The Community

For most people accountability is key, so you could start this programme with a friend or family member or join the Live Well group on Facebook. Here you can surround yourself with like-minded people, learn about the things that helped them and how they overcame obstacles. I'll also be there to motivate you, cheer you on and answer your questions.

Join The Group

https://www.facebook.com/groups/643942353656666

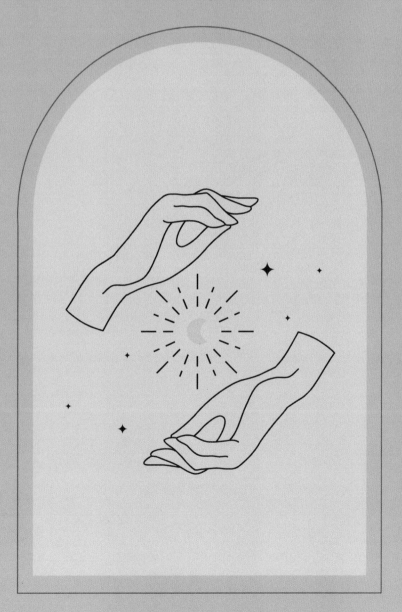

30 Day Action Plan

Before the start of each week, you'll be meal prepping - these are your meals for the week ahead. You'll also book time to workout for 45-minutes, 5 days a week, whilst maintaining a good sleep routine. The below are daily prompts and not replacements for the diet, exercise and sleep habits outlined.

01 ☐ Day 1! You planned your workouts and meal prepped. You can do this!	**02** ☐ Use the habit tracker to make sure you are on track with your diet, exercise & sleep	**03** ☐ Check in with your workouts and ensure you can fit in 5 workouts this week	**04** ☐ Review the next 25 days and assess if there will be any challenges. Plan for this	**05** ☐ If you haven't yet, join the Facebook group (page 89) and post about your progress
06 ☐ Meal prep following the checklist (page 34) ensuring plenty of variety	**07** ☐ Reflect on how the previous days went and what needs adjusting	**08** ☐ Assess and, if needed, optimise your bedtime routine	**09** ☐ Invite a friend to workout with you this week or join a class together	**10** ☐ Focus on your hydration - plan to drink 2L of water everyday
11 ☐ If it's been challenging remind yourself of why you're doing this programme	**12** ☐ Try a different workout class or increase your reps/workout time next week	**13** ☐ Experiment with different meals whilst following the format you've learnt about in Chapter 2	**14** ☐ Reflect on how the previous days went and what needs adjusting	**15** ☐ Use the Assessment on page 97 to check in with how you're feeling
16 ☐ Experiment with a workout that combines both movement and breath such as yoga or Tai Chi	**17** ☐ If you're not doing this already, experiment with meditating every night before bed	**18** ☐ Reflect on the parts of the programme that are bringing you joy	**19** ☐ Start focusing on eating intuitively and following your hunger cues	**20** ☐ Assess how you can optimise your meal prep technique to improve efficiency
21 ☐ Reflect on how the previous days went and what needs adjusting	**22** ☐ Introduce new workouts to your routine this week	**23** ☐ Share your progress and challenges in the Facebook group (page 89)	**24** ☐ Schedule time to get some sunlight in the morning - this will help your sleep	**25** ☐ On your rest days, think about how you can still find a little movement e.g. by walking instead of driving
26 ☐ Write down the foods that you used to like but don't tempt you anymore	**27** ☐ Experiment with different meals whilst following the format you've learnt about in Chapter 2	**28** ☐ Plan the next weeks as if you're still in The Programme	**29** ☐ Work on your mindset - strive for balance, not perfection	**30** ☐ **You did it!!!! Reward yourself to celebrate**

Live Well Habit Tracker
Week 1

This tracker summarises some important habits covered in the previous chapters. Aim to complete weekly to keep yourself accountable and monitor your progress so you know where to focus your attention.

Eat Well

		M	T	W	T	F	S	S
•	Meals reflect The Plate (page 15)	○	○	○	○	○	○	○
•	Avoid highly processed, high sugar foods	○	○	○	○	○	○	○
•	Drink at least 2 litres of water	○	○	○	○	○	○	○

Move Well

		M	T	W	T	F	S	S
•	45-minutes exercise (aim to tick 5 days)	○	○	○	○	○	○	○
•	Walk (at least for 10-minutes) on your rest days	○	○	○	○	○	○	○
•	Include stretches within your workout time	○	○	○	○	○	○	○

Sleep Well

		M	T	W	T	F	S	S
•	Enjoy your wind down routine	○	○	○	○	○	○	○
•	Sleep 7 - 9 hours per night	○	○	○	○	○	○	○
•	Meditate for 10 minutes	○	○	○	○	○	○	○

Live Well Habit Tracker
Week 2

This tracker summarises some important habits covered in the previous chapters. Aim to complete weekly to keep yourself accountable and monitor your progress so you know where to focus your attention.

Eat Well

	M	T	W	T	F	S	S
Meals reflect The Plate (page 15)	●	●	●	●	●	●	●
Avoid highly processed, high sugar foods	●	●	●	●	●	●	●
Drink at least 2 litres of water	●	●	●	●	●	●	●

Move Well

	M	T	W	T	F	S	S
45-minutes exercise (aim to tick 5 days)	●	●	●	●	●	●	●
Walk (at least for 10-minutes) on your rest days	●	●	●	●	●	●	●
Include stretches within your workout time	●	●	●	●	●	●	●

Sleep Well

	M	T	W	T	F	S	S
Enjoy your wind down routine	●	●	●	●	●	●	●
Sleep 7 - 9 hours per night	●	●	●	●	●	●	●
Meditate for 10 minutes	●	●	●	●	●	●	●

Live Well Habit Tracker
Week 3

This tracker summarises some important habits covered in the previous chapters. Aim to complete weekly to keep yourself accountable and monitor your progress so you know where to focus your attention.

Eat Well

M T W T F S S

- Meals reflect The Plate (page 15)

- Avoid highly processed, high sugar foods

- Drink at least 2 litres of water

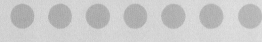

Move Well

M T W T F S S

- 45-minutes exercise (aim to tick 5 days)
- Walk (at least for 10-minutes) on your rest days
- Include stretches within your workout time

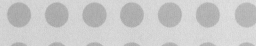

Sleep Well

M T W T F S S

- Enjoy your wind down routine

- Sleep 7 - 9 hours per night

- Meditate for 10 minutes

Live Well Habit Tracker
Week 4

This tracker summarises some important habits covered in the previous chapters. Aim to complete weekly to keep yourself accountable and monitor your progress so you know where to focus your attention.

Eat Well

	M	T	W	T	F	S	S
Meals reflect The Plate (page 15)	●	●	●	●	●	●	●
Avoid highly processed, high sugar foods	●	●	●	●	●	●	●
Drink at least 2 litres of water	●	●	●	●	●	●	●

Move Well

	M	T	W	T	F	S	S
45-minutes exercise (aim to tick 5 days)	●	●	●	●	●	●	●
Walk (at least for 10-minutes) on your rest days	●	●	●	●	●	●	●
Include stretches within your workout time	●	●	●	●	●	●	●

Sleep Well

	M	T	W	T	F	S	S
Enjoy your wind down routine	●	●	●	●	●	●	●
Sleep 7 - 9 hours per night	●	●	●	●	●	●	●
Meditate for 10 minutes	●	●	●	●	●	●	●

Weekly Planner

MON

TUE

WED

THU

FRI

SAT

SUN

MON

TUE

WED

THU

FRI

SAT

SUN

Check-In With Yourself

Before starting this programme you should have completed The Circle of Life on page 9. Use this scale to check in with how you're feeling with each area of the programme at days 15 and 30. Instead of focusing on your progress - you can use the Live Well Habit Tracker (pages 91 - 94) for that - consider your overall satisfaction. You form better habits when you enjoy them, so it's important that we look at your progress holistically. If your satisfaction with your diet, exercise or sleep has decreased, reflect on exactly what you're not happy with and make the necessary changes to improve it. If your satisfaction has increased, then keep going - you're doing amazing!

DAY 15

Diet

-4   -3   -2   -1   0   1   2   3   4

Exercise

-4   -3   -2   -1   0   1   2   3   4

Sleep

-4   -3   -2   -1   0   1   2   3   4

DAY 30

Diet

-4   -3   -2   -1   0   1   2   3   4

Exercise

-4   -3   -2   -1   0   1   2   3   4

Sleep

-4   -3   -2   -1   0   1   2   3   4

Thank You

Thank you for taking the time to read this book which I hope will be a turning point in your life. It would mean the world to me if you could please leave a review as this will help more people to discover this book. Thank you so much for your support.

If you want more recipes and wellness tips, subscribe to my monthly newsletter via my website manalivinghealing.com.

I'd love to hear from you, and how you got on with the programme, so please pop over to Instagram or Facebook to say hi!

References

1. Srivastava, RAK. Life-style-induced metabolic derangement and epigenetic changes promote diabetes and oxidative stress leading to NASH and atherosclerosis severity. J Diabetes Metab Disord. 2018 Dec; 17(2): 381–391.

2. Barrón-Cabrera, E et al. Epigenetic Modifications as Outcomes of Exercise Interventions Related to Specific Metabolic Alterations: A Systematic Review. Lifestyle Genom 2019;12(1-6):25-44.

3. Carden, L et al. Habit formation and change. Current Opinion in Behavioral Sciences Volume 20, April 2018, Pages 117-122.

4. Clear J. Atomic Habits: An Easy & Proven Way to Build Good Habits & Break Bad Ones. First Edition. London. Penguin Random House, 2018.

5. Quinn, JM et al. Can't Control Yourself? Monitor Those Bad Habits. Pers Soc Psychol Bull 2010; 36; 499.

6. Rubin G. Better Than Before: What I Learned About Making and Breaking Habits--to Sleep More, Quit Sugar, Procrastinate Less, and Generally Build a Happier Life. First Edition. New York. Penguin Random House LLC, 2015.

7. Greger M. How Not to Die: Discover the Foods Scientifically Proven to Prevent and Reverse Disease. London. Macmillan, 2016.

8. Wardle, J et al. Impact of stress on diet: Processes and implications. In S. A. Stansfeld & M. G. Marmot (Eds.), Stress and the heart: Psychosocial pathways to coronary heart disease (pp. 124–149). BMJ Books, 2002.

9. Ridder D et al. Healthy diet: Health impact, prevalence, correlates, and interventions. Psychology & Health 2017; 32:8, 907-941.

10. NHS Exercise Guidelines as of 4th August 2021.

11. Physical activity: applying All Our Health. Public Health England, Updated 16 October 2019.

12. New report assesses impact of physical inactivity on UK heart health and economy. British Heart Foundation, 3rd April 2017.

13. Jakicic, JM et al. Objective Physical Activity and Weight Loss in Adults: The Step-Up Randomized Clinical Trial. Obesity (Silver Spring). 2014 Nov; 22(11): 2284–2292.

14. Moreno-Agostino, D. et al. The impact of physical activity on healthy ageing trajectories: evidence from eight cohort studies. Int J Behav Nutr Phys Act. 2020; 17: 92.

15. Hwang, H. et al. Comparison of association between physical activity and resting metabolic rate in young and middle-aged Korean adults. J Exerc Nutrition Biochem. 2019 Jun 30; 23(2): 16–21.

References

16. Booth, FW. et al. Role of Inactivity in Chronic Diseases: Evolutionary Insight and Pathophysiological Mechanisms. Physiol Rev. 2017 Oct 1; 97(4): 1351–1402.

17. Kubala, AG. et al. The association between physical activity and a composite measure of sleep health. Sleep Breath. 2020 Sep; 24(3): 1207–1214.

18. Pizot, C. et al. Physical activity, hormone replacement therapy and breast cancer risk: A meta-analysis of prospective studies. Eur J Cancer. 2016 Jan;52:138-54.

19. Bull, FC. et al. World Health Organization 2020 guidelines on physical activity and sedentary behaviour. Br J Sports Med. 2020 Dec; 54(24): 1451–1462.

20. Banks, S. et al. Behavioral and Physiological Consequences of Sleep Restriction. J Clin Sleep Med. 2007 Aug 15; 3(5): 519–528.

21. Dashti, HS. Short Sleep Duration and Dietary Intake: Epidemiologic Evidence, Mechanisms, and Health Implications. Adv Nutr. 2015 Nov; 6(6): 648–659.

22. Report dated 2013, accessed via The Sleep Council website.

23. Hirshkowitz, M. et al. National Sleep Foundation's sleep time duration recommendations: methodology and results summary. Sleep Health. 2015 Mar;1(1):40-43.

24. Accessed via The Sleep Charity website.

25. Patel, AK. Physiology, Sleep Stages. Treasure Island (FL): StatPearls Publishing; January 2021.

26. Binks, H. et al. Effects of Diet on Sleep: A Narrative Review. Nutrients. 2020 Apr; 12(4): 936.

27. Walsh, JK et al. Effect of caffeine on physiological sleep tendency and ability to sustain wakefulness at night. Psychopharmacology (Berl). 1990;101(2):271-3.

28. Gao, Q. et al. The Association between Vitamin D Deficiency and Sleep Disorders: A Systematic Review and Meta-Analysis. Nutrients. 2018 Oct; 10(10): 1395.

29. Singh, NA. et al. A randomized controlled trial of the effect of exercise on sleep. Sleep. 1997 Feb;20(2):95-101.

30. Dobrosielski, DA. et al. Effects of exercise and weight loss in older adults with obstructive sleep apnea. Med Sci Sports Exerc. 2015 Jan;47(1):20-6.

31. Based on recommendations from The Sleep Charity, October 2021.

Printed in Great Britain
by Amazon

74746907R00058